A DENTAL PRACTITIONER HANDBOOK
SERIES EDITED BY DONALD D. DERRICK, D.D.S., L.D.S. R.C.S.

FRACTURES OF THE MANDIBLE

By

H. C. KILLEY

F.D.S. R.C.S.(Eng.), F.D.S., H.D.D. R.C.S.(Edin.),
L.R.C.P.(Lond.), M.R.C.S.(Eng.), F.I.C.S.

Professor of Oral Surgery, London University.
Head of Department of Oral Surgery,
Institute of Dental Surgery.
Hon. Consultant in Oral Surgery, Eastman Dental Hospital
and Westminster Hospital Teaching Group.
Formerly: Consultant in Oral Surgery and Maxillo-facial Injuries,
Plastic and Jaw Unit, Rooksdown House, Basingstoke,
Holy Cross Hospital, Haslemere,
Aldershot General Hospital,
and Queen Mary's Hospital, Roehampton

SECOND EDITION
REVISED REPRINT

BRISTOL: JOHN WRIGHT & SONS LTD.
1974

First Edition, 1967
Second Edition, 1971
Reprinted, 1974
Reprinted, 1977

By the same Author
Fractures of the Middle Third of the Facial Skeleton 2nd ed.
and with G. R. Seward and L. W. Kay
An Outline of Oral Surgery, Parts 1 and 2
Bristol: John Wright & Sons Ltd.

ISBN 0 7236 0395 2

PRINTED IN GREAT BRITAIN BY HENRY LING LTD. AT THE DORSET PRESS, DORCHESTER
A SUBSIDIARY OF JOHN WRIGHT AND SONS LTD.

PREFACE TO THE REVISED REPRINT

SINCE the Second Edition of this monograph was published in 1971 there have been no important advances in the interpretation of the surgical anatomy nor in the diagnosis of mandibular fractures, and the general principles of treatment are also unaltered. Only minimal revision of the main body of the text has therefore been necessary.

However, there is an increasing interest in bone plating and especially the use of compression bone plates and the section on this form of treatment has been expanded and important new references on the subject have been added to the bibliography. This is an interesting development but the present bone plating techniques have a number of serious disadvantages and internal fixation of mandibular fractures is unlikely to replace the more conventional forms of treatment in the immediate future.

July, 1974   H. C. K.

PREFACE TO THE FIRST EDITION

THIS outline of the diagnosis and treatment of fractures of the mandible is written as an introduction for students and as an aid to practitioners who treat mandibular fractures. It is not intended for the specialist maxillo-facial surgeon, for in a book of this size it is impossible to cover the subject in the necessary detail. Technical data on splint construction have been omitted for the same reason and only the more important aspects of the techniques for immobilization of the fragments have been discussed. The complex subject of the so-called 'gunshot-type' fracture where there is loss of both hard and soft tissues has of necessity been dealt with very briefly.

At the Editor's request, references have been reduced to a minimum in an endeavour to make the text easier to read and the author apologizes for many important omissions. However, mention has been made in the Bibliography of the many excellent articles and books which have been consulted.

It is important that all dental surgeons should be familiar with the diagnosis and treatment of mandibular fractures. Such injuries are easy to diagnose and after a careful examination the clinician can correlate the physical signs with the underlying surgical anatomy, so visualizing the nature and extent of the bony injury. Radiology, if available, should never be omitted, but in most instances the radiographs should merely confirm the clinical findings.

The treatment of the majority of mandibular fractures should be well within the capabilities of any dental surgeon, for provided the fracture is accurately reduced and adequately immobilized for the requisite period of time, a satisfactory result can be confidently expected. It is important to avoid infection of the fracture line during healing and for this reason it is helpful to begin a prophylactic course of antibiotics as soon after injury as possible and to continue this treatment until shortly after reduction and immobilization of the fracture. This avoids infection of the fracture haematoma, and experience has shown that it is much easier to prevent infection in this area than to treat an established infection. Reduction and immobilization should, of course, be effected as soon as the general medical condition of the patient permits.

H. C. K.

CONTENTS

ACKNOWLEDGEMENTS

My thanks are due to my secretary, Mrs. B. Rayiru, for much pains-taking work in typing this manuscript, to Mr. E. Warner for the diagrams, and to the Photographic Department of the Eastman Dental Hospital for the illustrations. My thanks are also due to Mr. Lester Kay, M.D.S., F.D.S., M.R.C.S., L.R.C.P., Reader in Oral Surgery at the Eastman Dental Hospital, for reading the script. I am indebted to the late Professor Aitchison and *The Dental Magazine* for permission to publish *Fig.* 15.

FRACTURES OF THE MANDIBLE

CHAPTER I

CLASSIFICATION

FRACTURES of the mandible may conveniently be divided into two main groups: (1) Fractures with no gross comminution of the bone and where there is no loss of hard or soft tissue; (2) Fractures with gross comminution of the bone and where there is extensive destruction of both hard and soft tissue.

Fractures of the first group, where there is no loss of hard or soft tissue, are often referred to as 'civilian-type' fractures, and the second group, where there is extensive destruction of both hard and soft tissue, is referred to as 'gunshot-type' fractures.

Although the expressions 'civilian' and 'gunshot' fracture are a convenient way of describing the injuries, it is, of course, possible to have a gunshot wound with minimal bony damage and no soft tissue loss, while some civilian-type injuries result in massive destruction of both the hard and soft tissues. The techniques used for immobilization of the bony fragments are common to both so-called 'civilian-' and 'gunshot-type' fractures, but the general management of the injury where there is hard and soft tissue loss is entirely different and treatment is inevitably protracted.

CIVILIAN-TYPE FRACTURES

Classification.—Fractures of the mandible may be simple, compound, comminuted, or pathological.

Fractures of the condyle, coronoid process, and ramus are usually simple, but fractures occurring in the tooth-bearing area of the mandible are often compound into the mouth or more rarely compound externally on the face.

Comminuted fractures occur following extreme violence or when a relatively sharp object has penetrated the tissues over the mandible and struck the bone violently. Such an object acts as a slow-moving missile, and may shatter both teeth and jaw.

Pathological fractures occur as a result of minimal trauma to a mandible already weakened by the presence of an osteomyelitic condition or a benign or malignant neoplasm (*Fig.* 1).

The greenstick fracture is a rare variant of the simple fracture which is found almost exclusively in children.

There is no completely satisfactory and generally accepted classification of mandibular fractures, but for purposes of diagnosis and treatment they may conveniently be considered under the following headings:—
1. Unilateral fracture.
2. Bilateral fracture.
3. Multiple fractures.
1. Unilateral Fracture.—Unilateral fractures are usually single, but occasionally more than one fracture may be present on one side of the

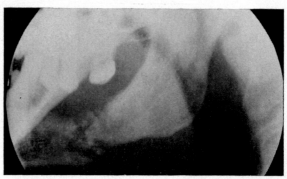

Fig. 1.—Pathological fracture of the mandible as a result of osteomyelitis following an extraction.

mandible and if this occurs there is usually gross displacement of the fragments. The single unilateral fracture is best described and classified according to the anatomical location of the injury, for the signs and symptoms vary according to the site of fracture as does the treatment. The following main types of fracture occur (*Fig.* 2):—
　a. Dento-alveolar.
　b. Condylar.
　c. Coronoid.
　d. Ramus.
　e. Angle.
　f. Body (molar and premolar area).
　g. Midline.
　h. Lateral to midline in the incisor region.
2. Bilateral Fracture.—Every possible combination and variation of the unilateral varieties of fracture already mentioned can occur bilaterally and these permutations will not be enumerated.
Possibly the most common bilateral fracture is the condylar neck fracture in association with a fracture of the opposite angle of the mandible. A canine region fracture together with a fracture of the opposite angle is also seen frequently, but, as already stated, any possible combination of fractures may occur.
3. Multiple Fractures.—When there are multiple fractures both sides of the jaw are usually affected and once again any possible combination of the fracture sites already described for the unilateral fracture may occur or the jaw may be comminuted.

The most common multiple fracture is the triple fracture which consists of a midline fracture of the mandible together with fractures of both condylar necks, which occurs if the patient falls heavily on the point of the chin, usually as a result of sudden loss of consciousness. These fractures are therefore commonly seen in epileptics, soldiers who faint on parade, and elderly patients who sustain a cerebral or cardiac catastrophe.

Oikarinen and Malmstrom (1969), in a series of 600 mandibular fractures, found 49·1 per cent had only a single fracture, 39·9 per cent had two fractures, 9·4 per cent had three fractures, 1·2 per cent had four fractures, and 0·4 per cent more than four fractures.

As already stated, extreme violence to the lower jaw or trauma from an object which penetrates the soft tissues and strikes the bone violently may result in comminution of the mandible to a greater or a lesser extent.

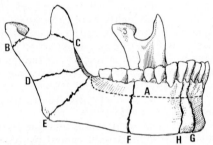

Fig. 2.—Classification of mandibular fracture sites: A, Dento-alveolar; B, Condylar; C, Coronoid; D, Ramus; E, Angle; F, Body; G, Midline; H, Lateral to midline in incisor area.

Common Sites of Fracture.—Unilateral fractures occur more frequently than bilateral or multiple fractures and the most common sites of unilateral fracture in their order of frequency are the neck of the condyle, the angle of the mandible, and the canine region. The occurrence of fractures in these particular areas may possibly be influenced by the following factors.

Fractures of the neck of the condyle are usually brought about by indirect violence. The patient receives a blow on the point of the chin and the force is directed backwards and upwards against the base of the skull. Very rarely this may result in the head of the condyle being driven through the glenoid fossa into the middle fossa of the skull, but fortunately this seldom occurs and usually the slender neck of the condyle fractures. Fracture of the neck of the condyle can therefore be regarded as a safety mechanism which protects the patient from the serious consequences of a middle fossa fracture.

There is a line of weakness at the angle of the mandible where the comparatively thin ramus joins the body of the mandible. The presence of an unerupted lower third molar may further weaken the jaw in this area. Fractures of the angle of the mandible may be produced by either direct or indirect violence.

The canine region is the site of election for intentional and unintentional direct violence and if a canine tooth is present the fact that its root is slightly longer than the neighbouring teeth may constitute a line of weakness.

Oikarinen and Malmstrom (1969) analysed 600 mandibular fractures in a most ingenious manner by taking tracings from orthopantomographs. These tracings were analysed and 33·4 per cent fractures were found in the subcondylar area, 17·4 per cent at the angle, 6·7 per cent were alveolar, 5·4 per cent were in the ramus, 2·9 per cent in the midline, and 1·3 per cent in the coronoid, while 33·6 per cent occurred in the body of the mandible, mostly in the canine region.

Aetiology.—Most civilian-type fractures of the mandible are caused through blows on the jaw sustained during the course of a fight, but any form of trauma to the mandible may result in a fracture.

Harnisch (1959), of the Rudolf Virchow Hospital, Berlin, analysed 532 fractures and found fights were responsible for 34·8 per cent. Lindstrom (1960), of Finland, in a series of 649 fractures, of which 84 per cent involved the mandible, found fights were responsible for 36·7 per cent. In a series of 871 mandibular fractures (Rowe and Killey, 1969) 239 or 27·43 per cent were caused by fights. Apart from fighting, almost any other form of trauma may cause a fracture of the mandible. Oikarinen and Malmstrom (1969), at the Institute of Dental Surgery, Helsinki, found that between 1945 and 1947 assault and battery was the predominant aetiological factor and 46 per cent of their jaw fractures were caused by such trauma. However, from 1958 to 1967 road traffic accidents became the most common cause of facial fractures and during this period 31 per cent of their maxillofacial injuries were caused by vehicle accidents and only 27 per cent were due to assault and battery.

Incidence.—Mandibular fractures are more common than middle third injuries. Schuchardt and others (1966), in their series of 2901 fractures, found 1947 involved the mandible alone while a further 156 cases involved both the mandible and the middle third of the facial skeleton, giving a total of 2103 mandibular fractures. Rowe and Killey (1969), in a series of 1500 fractures, found 871 involved the mandible alone and a further 128 affected both the mandible and the middle third, a total of 999 mandibular fractures. Oikarinen and Malmstrom (1969) analysed 1284 patients with fractures, of the jaw treated at the Institute of Dentistry, Helsinki, during a 10-year period. There were 958 involving the mandible and 101 the mandible and middle third, a total of 1059 mandibular fractures. Halazonetis (1968), in an analysis of 700 jaw fractures, found 465 occurred in the mandible alone, 140 in the middle third of the facial skeleton, and 95 involved both the mandible and middle third, a total of 560 mandibular fractures over a 12-year period 1951–63. However, Mallett (1950), who reviewed 2124 cases of facial fracture, stated that mandibular fractures were twenty times as common as middle third injuries.

CHAPTER II

CLINICAL EXAMINATION

THE examination of a patient with a fracture of the mandible should consist of:—
1. The general clinical examination of the patient;
2. The local examination of the mandibular fracture.

1. The General Clinical Examination of the Patient.—Fractures of the mandible are, of course, caused by trauma of varying degrees of severity and it is reasonable to consider the possibility that this trauma may also have caused injury elsewhere in the body. This is especially true if the patient has been involved in a severe accident such as a road traffic accident or a fall from a considerable height. However, a simple blow on the lower jaw as a result of a fight or during the course of some game may result in force being transmitted to the cranium which results in serious injury or even death of the patient. The mere fact that a patient is ambulant and apparently unaffected by the injury does not necessarily preclude the presence of more serious injury. Such a case seen by the author was a patient who sustained a simple crack fracture at the angle of the mandible during a game of Rugby football. The blow was not sufficient to cause loss of consciousness at the time of injury and the patient was ambulant when first seen and apparently in good health. Shortly after admission, however, the patient exhibited signs of cerebral haemorrhage and, in spite of neuro-surgical intervention, died the following day from a subarachnoid haemorrhage. Similar examples can be quoted from the statistics of fatalities following amateur and professional boxing injuries. It is imperative, therefore, that all traumatic cases should have a careful physical examination and no operative procedure should be carried out to treat a fracture until the operator is certain that the patient has not sustained an additional and more serious injury. Treatment of such an associated condition should, of course, take precedence over the mandibular fracture, but occasionally it may be treated concurrently. It should be remembered that elderly patients may fall and break their mandible as a result of a cerebral or cardiac catastrophe and this possibility must always be considered in such cases.

The most common associated injuries are cerebral haemorrhage, ruptured spleen, ruptured mesenteric arteries, haemothorax, ruptured kidneys, and fractured cervical spine or other bones. Failure to diagnose any of these injuries might result in a surgical disaster.

Fortunately, most major injuries are fairly obvious and careful inspection and gentle palpation of the unclothed body in a good light will usually reveal their presence. It is unusual for a patient with a mandibular fracture to be shocked and if this condition is present some more serious injury should be suspected.

2. The Local Examination of the Mandibular Fracture.—Before carrying out a careful clinical examination of the mandibular fracture, the face should be gently cleaned with warm water or swabs to remove caked blood, road dirt, etc., so as to enable an accurate evaluation to be made of any soft tissue lacerations and associated ecchymosis. Similarly, the mouth should be examined for loose or broken teeth or dentures, and any congealed blood should be removed with swabs held in untoothed forceps. If a denture is fractured, the fragments should be assembled to make certain that no portion is missing—possibly displaced down the throat. Only after careful cleaning has been carried out extra- and intra-orally is it possible to evaluate accurately the extent of the injury.

It is surprising how the apparent magnitude of the surgical problem diminishes as the overlying blood is removed and accurate visualization becomes possible. When the gentle cleaning of the face is completed the cranium and cervical spine are carefully inspected and then gently palpated for signs of injury, after which the mandibular fracture is examined.

Clinical Examination of Mandibular Fracture.—

On inspection extra-orally: Over the site of the fracture there is usually ecchymosis and swelling. Often there is an associated soft tissue laceration and there may be obvious deformity of the bony contour of the mandible. If considerable displacement of the fragments has occurred, the patient is unable to close the anterior teeth together properly and the mouth hangs slackly open, the patient often finding it more comfortable to support the lower jaw with his hand. Most mandibular fractures are compound into the mouth, and as this usually results in haemorrhage, blood-stained saliva may be seen dribbling from the corner of the mouth in patients with a recent fracture. Patients usually have a characteristic unhappy, worried, hurt expression.

On palpation extra-orally: Gentle palpation with the tips of the fingers should be made over the condylar region bilaterally and then continued downwards along the lower border of the mandible.

Tenderness will be detected over the fracture sites and it may be possible to feel step defects in the bone, alteration in bony contour, or bony crepitus.

If the fracture involves the mandibular nerve, there will be anaesthesia of the lower lip over the mental distribution of the nerve, and the physical sign should be elicited at this stage of the examination.

On inspection intra-orally: Firstly, any portions of broken teeth or dentures should be removed from the mouth if this has not already been carried out. It is impossible to assess intra-oral damage if the parts are obscured by blood. If the patient is conscious and ambulant, a mouthwash of cold water is helpful, but in most cases the clinician will have to remove the clotted blood by gently cleaning the area with swabs. Congealed blood can be peeled off teeth with untoothed forceps and then any loose portions of teeth or alveolus are gently lifted out of the mouth. The area is examined in a good light.

First, the buccal sulcus is inspected for ecchymosis and after this the lingual sulcus is examined for ecchymosis or the presence of a fracture haematoma. Ecchymosis in the buccal sulcus is not necessarily indicative of a mandibular fracture for there is considerable soft tissue overlying the bone in this area and extensive ecchymosis may arise following a blow over the lower jaw which does not result in fracture. However, on the lingual side the mucosa of the floor of the mouth overlies the periosteum of the mandible and ecchymosis or haematoma in the lingual sulcus following trauma to the lower jaw is almost pathognomonic of a mandibular fracture (*Fig.* 3).

Next, the occlusal plane of the teeth is examined or, if the patient is edentulous, the alveolar ridge. Step defects in the occlusion or alveolus

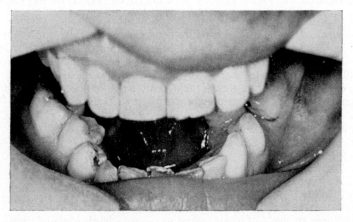

Fig. 3.—Haematoma in floor of mouth as a result of a mandibular fracture.

are noted as are any obvious lacerations in the overlying mucosa, which are often indicative of an underlying fracture. Obvious fracture, luxation, or subluxation of the teeth are noted, as are any missing crowns, bridges, or fillings. If teeth, portions of teeth, dentures, fillings, etc., are missing a note is made to order a radiograph of the chest in case they have been inhaled.

On palpation intra-orally: The lingual and buccal sulci are gently palpated and a note is made of areas of tenderness and step deformities in the bone. Each tooth present is gently tested for mobility and other signs of fracture or subluxation. Suspected fracture sites are noted and the thumb and forefinger of each hand are placed either side of the possible fracture site and gentle pressure is used to elicit unnatural mobility across the site of fracture.

Lastly, if the patient can co-operate, he is asked to carry out a full range of mandibular movements and any pain or limitation in movement is observed. Finally, all teeth in the mouth should be carefully examined with a mirror and probe to detect loose fillings, fine cracks, or splits in the tooth substance.

CHAPTER III

SIGNS, SYMPTOMS, AND SURGICAL ANATOMY OF MANDIBULAR FRACTURES ACCORDING TO THE SITES OF FRACTURE

THE signs and symptoms of fracture occurring in the different regions of the mandible vary according to the surgical anatomy of the area involved, and it is therefore helpful to consider the signs and symptoms of mandibular fractures together with the associated surgical anatomy.

As already stated, fractures of the mandible can be divided according to their anatomical location into eight main types. These are:—

A, Dento-alveolar
B, Condylar
C, Coronoid
D, Ramus
E, Angle
F, Body (molar and premolar area)
G, Midline
H, Lateral to midline in the incisor area.

Fractures in each of these situations have clearly defined signs and symptoms which can be readily elicited even in cases of multiple injury.

A. DENTO-ALVEOLAR FRACTURES

Dento-alveolar injuries consist of avulsion, subluxation, or fracture of the teeth with or without an associated alveolar fracture and they may occur alone or in conjunction with any other type of mandibular fracture.

Damage to the Teeth.—One of the most common injuries following trauma to the lower jaw is damage to the crown of a tooth which may fracture with or without exposure of the pulp chamber. Sometimes the injury forces the soft tissues of the lip against the lower incisor teeth, producing a ragged laceration on its inner aspect or possibly a full-thickness wound. Frequently such an injury smashes the crown of one or more teeth and portions of these teeth may be embedded in the lower lip.

Fractures of the roots of teeth may occur and these are often comminuted beneath the gum. A fractured crown or a completely avulsed tooth may possibly be inhaled by the patient at the time of accident and if a tooth or portion of tooth is missing it is always desirable to have a radiograph of the patient's chest, especially if there was loss of consciousness at the time of injury. Subluxation of one or more teeth leads to mobility and displacement of the teeth concerned and derangement of the occlusion.

Alveolar Fracture.—Fractures of the alveolus may be caused with or without associated injuries of the teeth. Gross comminution of the alveolus occurs following severe trauma, but usually a single alveolar fragment is present (*Figs.* 4, 5).

Clinical Examination of Dento-alveolar Fractures.—On inspection there may be a full-thickness wound of the lower lip or a ragged laceration is seen on its inner aspect. There is usually oedema and ecchymosis of the lip.

On examining the teeth and alveolus there may be lacerations, ecchymosis of the gum, and deformity of the alveolus. Teeth may be missing and the presence of a recent extraction wound suggests that the tooth has been knocked out. The remaining teeth may be mobile, subluxated, or fractured. Occasionally the molar teeth appear normal, but careful examination reveals that they are split vertically as a result of being violently

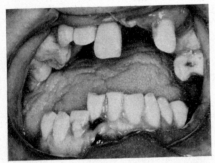

Fig. 4.—Alveolar fracture involving 1|12345. The patient reported to a dental surgeon several days after the injury and insisted that the painful 3 should be extracted. On applying forceps to this tooth the 1|12345 also moved.

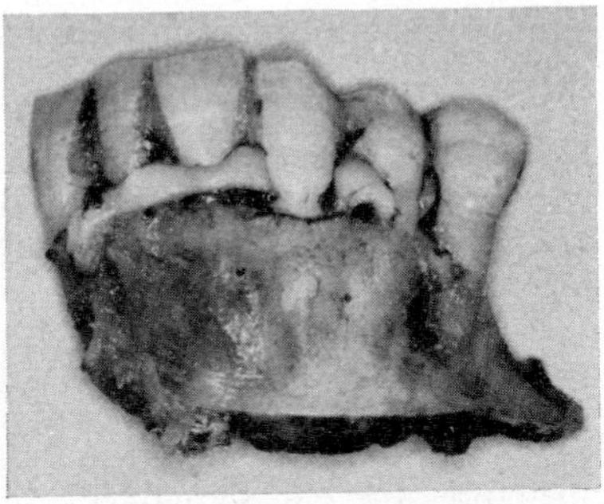

Fig. 5.—The alveolar fracture shown in Fig. 4 was heavily infected and the fragment had to be removed.

impacted against the upper molars and premolars. Often several teeth are damaged in this manner and careful inspection of the occlusal surfaces of the teeth with a mirror and probe is required to detect this type of injury.

On Palpation.—Gentle palpation of the lip may reveal the presence of teeth or portions of their crowns embedded in the tissues. Gentle palpation of the alveolus will reveal bony deformity and even crepitus, if comminution of the alveolus has occurred. Teeth are gently tested for mobility and vitality tests are carried out on all damaged teeth to gauge their viability. An interesting intra-oral split in the soft tissues overlying the bone sometimes occurs parallel to the gingival margin when a patient is flung onto the point of the chin as a result of an accident and lands on some resilient substance such as soft earth. The jaw does not fracture but the soft tissue is violently rotated over the point of the chin and the tissues tear at the junction of the attached and free gingivae in a line parallel to the gingival margin.

B. CONDYLAR FRACTURES

This is the most common fracture of the mandible and it may easily fail to be detected on casual examination.

Condylar fractures can be classified as intracapsular and extracapsular and unilateral or bilateral. Intracapsular fractures are rare, but the extracapsular fractures of the condylar neck are probably the most common mandibular fracture. The extracapsular fracture may exist with or without dislocation of the condylar head and the upper fragment may either be angulated on the lower portion of the ramus or it may be displaced buccally or lingually. Angulation is due to the pull of the external pterygoid which is attached to the antromedial aspect of the condylar head.

In the immediate post-traumatic phase most fractures in the condylar area exhibit similar signs and symptoms.

Unilateral Condylar Fracture.—

Clinical Examination.—

On inspection: On inspection extra-orally there is swelling over the temporomandibular joint area and there may be haemorrhage from the ear on that side.

Usually the bleeding is from a small split in the skin on the anterior aspect of the external auditory meatus. This occurs as the condylar head is pulled violently away from beneath the skin where it can be felt moving in the normal subject if the little finger is hooked into the external auditory meatus.

If the condylar head has been pushed through the glenoid fossa into the middle fossa of the skull and if there is a middle fossa fracture, severe bleeding may occur from the ear and there will probably be an associated cerebrospinal fluid otorrhoea. In all cases of suspected condylar fracture, therefore, the ear should be examined carefully, especially if there is haemorrhage from this area. If the condylar head is dislocated and all oedema has subsided due to passage of time, it may be possible to observe the characteristic hollow over the condylar head region, but in the immediate post-traumatic phase this physical sign is obscured by oedema.

On palpation: Palpation in the recently injured patient will elicit tenderness over the condylar area. When post-traumatic oedema is present it is impossible to detect movement of the condylar head on palpation and what is believed to be the condylar head may, in fact, be that portion of the fractured condylar neck attached to the lower portion of the ramus.

However, when all oedema has subsided it may be possible to decide whether the condylar head is within the glenoid fossa and whether it is moving with the remainder of the mandible. Standing in front of the patient both little fingers should be hooked into the external auditory meatus and movement of both condylar heads can then be compared and clicking or crepitation can also be determined. Haemorrhage in the condylar head region may track across the base of the skull and exert pressure on the mandibular division of the 5th cranial nerve as it emerges from the foramen ovale. This may cause anaesthesia of the lower lip and if present this physical sign should be elicited.

On inspection intra-orally: There will be a deviation of the occlusion towards the fractured side and this is especially obvious when the patient opens the mouth. When mandibular movement is tested lateral excursion towards the fractured side can be effected without much discomfort, but lateral excursion to the opposite side is limited and painful. Mandibular protrusion is also limited and painful.

Bilateral Condylar Fractures.—

Extra-orally.—

The signs and symptoms on inspection and palpation already mentioned for the unilateral fracture may be present on both sides.

On Inspection Intra-orally.—

On intra-oral examination the bilateral condylar fractures can be divided into two main groups: those where the occlusion is not deranged and those with an anterior open bite. Specialized and protracted treatment is required for the latter group. In both varieties there is pain and limitation on opening and there is pain and limitation on attempted lateral excursion or protrusion of the mandible.

Bilateral condylar fractures are frequently associated with a midline fracture of the mandible and the incisor area of the mandible should be examined carefully for a crack fracture in such cases.

C. Fracture of the Coronoid Process

This is a rare fracture which is said to be brought about by muscular pull and if the tip of the coronoid process is detached the fragment is pulled upwards towards the infratemporal fossa by the temporalis muscle (*Fig.* 6).

The coronoid process is sometimes fractured during operations on large cysts of the ramus or when removing impacted lower third molars which

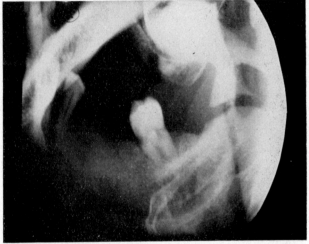

Fig. 6.—Lateral oblique radiograph showing fracture of the coronoid process with displacement due to pull of temporalis muscle.

have assumed an aberrant position in the area of the coronoid process. It is a difficult fracture to diagnose with certainty on clinical examination, but intra-orally there may be some ecchymosis in the area and tenderness on palpation over the region of the coronoid process. There may be pain and limitation of mandibular movement especially on protrusion of the mandible.

D. Fracture of the Ramus

Fractures confined to the ramus are rare and there are two main types:—

1. A Single Fracture across the Ramus.—This may also be regarded as a very low extracapsular condylar fracture, with both the coronoid process and condylar neck and head on the upper fragment.

2. A Comminuted Fracture of the Ramus.—The fragments in such fractures are splinted between the masseter and the internal pterygoid muscles and little displacement occurs unless there has been extreme violence.

Clinical Examination.—On extra-oral and intra-oral inspection there may be some swelling and ecchymosis. Palpation produces tenderness over the ramus both extra- and intra-orally and mandibular movements produce pain over the area.

DISPLACEMENT OF FRAGMENTS IN FRACTURES OF THE ANGLE AND BODY OF THE MANDIBLE

The displacement of the fragments of bone following fracture at the angle and through the body of the mandible depends on the site of the fracture, the direction of the fracture lines through the bone, and the pull on the muscles attached to the fragments.

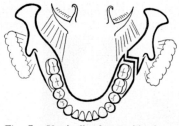

Fig. 7.—Vertically favourable fracture at the left angle of the mandible.

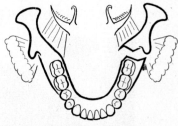

Fig. 8.—Vertically unfavourable fracture at the left angle of the mandible.

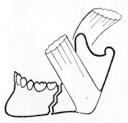

Fig. 9.—Horizontally favourable fracture at the angle of the mandible.

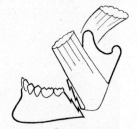

Fig. 10.—Horizontally unfavourable fracture at the angle of the mandible.

E. FRACTURES AT THE ANGLE

After fractures of the condylar neck, this is the most common mandibular fracture.

An arbitrary classification of favourable or unfavourable fracture is made in this region depending upon whether the posterior fragment is grossly displaced. The displacement is caused by the pull of the masseter and/or the internal pterygoid, and the degree of displacement depends upon the direction of the fracture line vertically and horizontally through the bone.

If the vertical direction of the fracture line favours the unopposed action of the internal pterygoid muscle the posterior fragment will be pulled lingually, and if the horizontal direction of the fracture line favours the unopposed action of the masseter and internal pterygoid muscle in an upward direction the posterior fragment will be displaced upwards. Fractures in this area may therefore be favourable or unfavourable in a vertical or horizontal direction, as seen in *Figs. 7–10*.

It should be remembered, however, that favourable and/or unfavourable fracture lines in a horizontal and vertical direction coexist. Either may result in impaction of the bone ends with minimal displacement, or the posterior fragment may be dragged into an abnormal position. From a practical point of view, if the fracture is relatively stable it is considered a favourable fracture irrespective of the apparent direction of the lines of fracture.

Extreme violence will displace the posterior fragment in spite of a favourable line of fracture. However, on reduction of such a fracture the favourable fracture line will assist the immobilization by preventing displacement.

The presence of an erupted tooth on the posterior fragment will limit gross displacement of the posterior fragment in an upward direction if its crown impacts on the opposing upper teeth. The presence of such a tooth will, of course, aid the subsequent reduction and immobilization of such a fragment.

F. FRACTURES OF THE BODY OF THE MANDIBLE (MOLAR AND PREMOLAR AREA)

Little displacement of the fragments occurs in a unilateral fracture of the body of the mandible in the molar and premolar areas as the muscles on either side of the fracture site tend to counteract each other. Fibres of the mylohyoid on either side of the fracture line probably play an important part in minimizing the displacement in this type of fracture.

G. FRACTURES IN THE MIDLINE OF THE MANDIBLE

Fractures in the midline of the mandible exhibit minimal displacement as the fracture line runs between the genial tubercles, and the pull of the geniohyoid and the genioglossus muscles tends to impact the bone ends together (*Fig. 11*). Such fractures are by no means uncommon and are seen in the so-called 'parade ground' or 'epileptic-type' injury sustained from a fall on the point of the chin. Sometimes the displacement of the fragments is so minimal that the fracture may be overlooked. Occasionally such a fracture is not readily apparent on an occlusal radiograph across the suspected fracture site, but an oblique occlusal radiograph will readily demonstrate the fracture. The presence of such a fracture should be suspected in all cases where a patient has fallen on the point of the chin and where bilateral condylar fractures are present.

H. FRACTURES IMMEDIATELY TO ONE SIDE OF THE MIDLINE

A fracture running to one side of the genial tubercles will exhibit considerable displacement as the muscles attached to the genial tubercles will tend to pull the greater fragment lingual to the lesser fragment.

Occasionally this is prevented by the direction of the fracture line vertically through the bone, but usually, even though there is a favourable line of fracture, the initial trauma will implement the displacement (*Fig.* 12). The most common site for such fractures is the canine area.

Signs and Symptoms of Fractures of Angle and Body of the Mandible.— The clinical findings in fractures of the angle and body of the mandible vary according to the site of the fracture. Certain signs and symptoms are, however, common to all fractures in this area.

*On Inspection.—*There is obvious deformity of the mandible and extra- and intra-oral oedema and ecchymosis occur with or without an associated soft tissue laceration.

There is a derangement of the occlusion or deformity of the alveolus if the patient is edentulous.

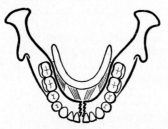

Fig. 11.—Fracture in the midline of the mandible. Minimal displacement occurs in such injuries as the fracture line passes between the genial tubercles.

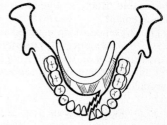

Fig. 12.—Fracture lateral to the midline in the incisor area. The fragment with the genial tubercles is displaced lingually by the pull of the geniohyoid and genioglossus muscles.

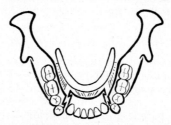

Fig. 13.—Bilateral fracture of the body of the mandible. The anterior fragment is displaced backwards by the pull of the muscles attached to the genial tubercles.

*On Palpation.—*There is tenderness on palpation in the region of the fracture and unnatural mobility can usually be elicited on gentle pressure across the fracture site, unless the fragments are tightly impacted.

If the mandibular nerve is involved there is anaesthesia of the lower lip in the mental distribution of the nerve. Depending on the site of the fracture the fragments are displaced in the manner already described.

*Movements.—*There is pain on attempted movement of the mandible and if any movement can be achieved it is limited in extent.

BILATERAL AND COMMINUTED FRACTURES

1. Bilateral Fractures of the Mandible.—As already stated, every possible permutation of the unilateral fracture can occur bilaterally. In general, the displacement seen in such fractures is more marked than in the unilateral fracture and this is especially true of the bilateral fracture of the body of the mandible (*Fig.* 13). Under these circumstances the pull of the muscles attached to the genial tubercles tends to pull back the anterior fragment and this results in a backward displacement of the tongue which is deprived of its anterior skeletal support. In such circumstances there may be a risk of respiratory embarrassment but this is more likely to occur with a comminuted fracture in the mental area (*Fig.* 14). In some cases the direction of the fracture lines through the bone precludes the backward displacement of the anterior fragment and it is tilted due to the pull of the muscles attached to the genial tubercles. This results in the lower teeth being displaced forwards and biting outside the upper incisors.

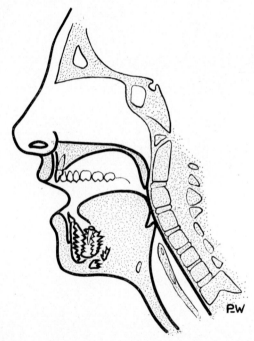

Fig. 14.—Midline comminuted fracture of the mandible involving the genial tubercles. The tongue has been deprived of its anterior skeletal attachment and has fallen back and is obstructing the airway.

2. Comminuted Fractures.—As already stated, comminuted fractures are either caused by extreme violence or are due to a relatively sharp object striking the bone and acting as a missile. Such injuries are often associated with a through-and-through wound. Comminuted fractures of the body of the mandible produce considerable displacement of the fragments and if they occur in the chin region the skeletal support of the tongue is destroyed and respiratory embarrassment will occur due to backward displacement of the tongue.

Clinical Findings of Bilateral and Comminuted Fractures.—The physical signs of bilateral and comminuted fractures depend on the site and number of the fractures and consist of combinations and permutations of the physical signs already discussed for the unilateral mandibular fracture. The symptoms are also similar to those found in the unilateral fracture but vary in severity according to the magnitude of the injury.

CHAPTER IV

RADIOLOGY

THE radiographs required for an examination of a fractured mandible are:—
1. Left and right oblique lateral.
2. Postero-anterior.
3. Periapical, intra-oral of teeth either side of fracture line.
4. Occlusal and possibly oblique occlusal across the fracture line.
5. Modified reverse Towne's.
Further Films which may be Necessary:—
6. Temporomandibular joint views.
7. Tomograms of the condylar head.
Oblique Lateral Radiographs:—
1. The oblique lateral radiographs should be centred over the suspected area of fracture and besides showing the body of the mandible and angle they may reveal a fracture of the condylar neck.
Postero-anterior Radiographs:—
2. The postero-anterior film demonstrates fractures of the body and angle together with the type of displacement. It is impossible to see the condylar head in a normal postero-anterior view as it is obscured by the superimposition of the mastoid process, and if it is visible it is strong presumptive evidence that a fracture is present.
Intra-oral Radiographs:—
3. Intra-oral periapical films are required to demonstrate whether teeth are involved in the fracture line.
4. Occlusal films across the fracture line help to evaluate the relation of the tooth root to the fracture line. They are also invaluable for demonstrating midline fractures with minimal displacement. If a midline fracture is suspected but cannot satisfactorily be demonstrated on the occlusal film an oblique occlusal will usually demonstrate the injury.
Reverse Towne's Views:—
5. The reverse Towne's is used to demonstrate a fracture of the condylar neck, as this cannot be accurately visualized in the postero-anterior view.
Temporomandibular Joint Views:—
6. Temporomandibular joint films with the mouth in the open and the closed position will demonstrate whether a dislocation is present and if the temporomandibular joint is functioning normally.
Tomograms:—
7. Tomography is helpful to demonstrate an intracapsular fracture and frequently this is the only radiograph which will reveal this type of injury.

- *Orthopantomograms:*—

8. The orthopantomogram is especially valuable in detecting mandibular fractures in the condylar region and it will occasionally demonstrate injuries which cannot be seen in the reverse Towne's views. Oikarinen and Malmstrom (1969) describe a useful method of recording mandibular fractures by making tracings of an orthopantomogram and copying the tracings onto a master copy. A record of the incidence, direction, and site of any given series of fractures can be accurately recorded in this fashion.

The radiographs should be taken by a radiographer who is experienced in maxillo facial work so as to ensure that the patient is not subjected to unnecessary discomfort. The radiological examination must be carried out with minimal manipulation of the affected mandible and the use of a special skull unit, such as a Schönander or a Barazzetti Skull Unit, is very helpful in this respect.

CHAPTER V

PRELIMINARY TREATMENT

First Aid.—Patients with a civilian-type fracture of the mandible, which is not associated with other more serious injury elsewhere in the body, seldom require first aid solely for the mandibular fracture. It is unusual for such patients to be shocked, nor is there excessive haemorrhage, but occasionally with bilateral fractures in the mental region the skeletal support of the tongue is lost and the tongue tends to be pulled backwards, so impeding respiration. In such cases a tongue stitch may be required and until such time as this is inserted the patient should be positioned so that the tongue does not fall back. To achieve this the unconscious patient should lie either face downwards or with the head on one side, while the sitting or ambulant patient should hold the head downwards and forwards. These positions also allow blood and saliva to dribble out of the mouth. As soon as practicable, the anterior fragment with its attached genial tubercles should be repositioned and immobilized with a definitive fixation such as an arch bar, etc., so stabilizing the tongue once more.

The mouth should always be carefully examined and any portions of broken denture, loose or fractured teeth and fillings, etc., should be removed to prevent them becoming inhaled. In most cases temporary splinting of the fragments is unnecessary and such devices as the barrel bandage, webbing head cap with elastic chin support, and Elastoplast chin strap are not only unnecessary but may in some instances cause the patient additional discomfort. If this type of first aid has been applied it is salutary to observe how often the patient experiences relief when it is removed. Usually, if any urgent immobilization of the fragment is required it is best to carry out a definitive standard fixation technique such as an arch bar or eyelet wiring, etc., and not to waste time with an ineffective temporary fixation.

Owing to the pain, conscious patients usually take good care not to move the fragments unnecessarily and often assist immobilization by supporting the lower jaw with their hands.

Antibiotic therapy such as 1 mega unit of procaine fortified penicillin daily should be started as soon as possible and oral hygiene measures such as mouth irrigation should be instituted.

Soft Tissue Lacerations.—If there are associated soft tissue lacerations these must be closed within 24 hours to avoid infection and if the operation for the reduction and immobilization of the fracture has to be deferred the soft tissue lacerations can be sutured under local analgesia.

Before closing wounds they must be carefully cleaned to remove road dirt, tar, etc., which will leave an ugly tattoo mark in the scar.

Cleansing of the wounds can be effected with Cetavlon 1 per cent and the use of a sterile soft toothbrush is helpful for this purpose.

Food and Fluid.—Food and fluid should, of course, be withheld if an immediate operation under general anaesthesia is contemplated, otherwise sips of fluid (soup) can be given using a feeding cup with a rubber-tube attachment. A fluid balance chart should be started and kept until such time as the patient is stabilized on a satisfactory fluid intake.

Sedation.—Patients with a mandibular fracture experience little pain and sedation is seldom necessary. It should be remembered that the use of powerful analgesics such as morphine are contra-indicated as they depress the cough reflex and respiratory centre and also mask pain which can be diagnostically important (i.e., as from an associated ruptured spleen or peritonitis). There is also the risk of a heavily sedated patient with a severe mandibular fracture dying as a result of respiratory obstruction from the tongue falling back or from blood in the trachea.

Transportation.—It is essential that patients with severe maxillofacial injuries are not laid on their back as they may rapidly develop respiratory obstruction and die. This is especially liable to occur in the case of comminuted mandibular fractures when the anterior skeletal support of the tongue is involved. Such patients should be transported lying on their side in a position which allows the tongue to fall forward and secretions to dribble out of the mouth. A tongue stitch should be inserted and a nurse should be in attendance during the journey. A portable sucker must be available.

CHAPTER VI

DEFINITIVE TREATMENT OF FRACTURES IN THE CONDYLAR REGION

SOME controversy exists concerning the most satisfactory method of treating fractures in the condylar region of the mandible and there are three main schools of thought on the subject. These are:—

1. Immobilization for a short period, i.e., about 7 days, in order to relieve pain and restore centric occlusion. This is followed by active mobilization of the mandible.

2. Encouragement of early movement as soon after the injury as possible.

3. Open reduction of the fracture and transosseous wiring of the fragments.

Each of these methods has ardent and enthusiastic advocates and excellent results are claimed for each of the techniques. There are, however, certain factors to be taken into consideration when deciding upon the most suitable treatment for these fractures.

Temporary Immobilization.—Immobilization of the injured joint for a short period (i.e., about 7 days) restores normal occlusion and rests the fractured area, so relieving pain. If this is followed by active mobilization of the mandible an excellent result is obtained.

Early Movement.—A similar result can be achieved by encouraging early movement without first carrying out a temporary immobilization of the mandible. Deviation of the mandible is usually due to painful muscle spasm and as soon as this wears off the patient assumes a normal occlusion.

Transosseous Wiring.—Transosseous wiring requires an external approach to the mandible and this will, of course, leave a scar no matter how skilful the operator. The surgical approach to the condylar region is from a pre-auricular or a submandibular incision. The operation is not easy as a high standard of surgical skill is required to avoid damage to the facial nerve or maxillary artery. Recently it has been shown by Walker (1960), following experimental work on Macaca monkeys, that the results following condylar fracture for all three forms of treatment were essentially similar. In this country transosseous wiring of the fractured condylar region is not employed as a routine treatment and operation on the condyle following fracture is usually reserved for cases of bony ankylosis following for instance an intracapsular fracture.

Pain following a condylar fracture rapidly subsides and as the patient tends to rest the mandible at this time active immobilization is usually unnecessary. It is unusual for the operator to have to resort to active immobilization to restore normal centric occlusion, but all condylar fracture patients should be kept under observation to ensure that a satisfactory occlusion is being achieved. Immediate mobilization of the mandible is the most simple form of treatment and as the results are exceptionally good it seems reasonable to advocate this method.

Immobilization for Periods Longer than 10 Days.—If the mandible is immobilized for a longer period than about 10 days there is a risk of bony union occurring with the condylar head in such a position that thereafter only limited movement is possible at that joint. In order to open the mouth the patient must subluxate the opposite joint so producing an ugly deviation of the mandible towards the side originally injured. For this reason immobilization should never be maintained beyond a week or 10 days. It used to be thought that in cases of fracture dislocation a pseudarthrosis resulted, but MacGregor and Fordyce, in 1957, showed a case of marked bilateral fracture dislocation of the mandible where bony union had occurred. In Walker's (1960) excellent paper on experimental condylar fractures in Macaca monkeys bony union occurred following fracture dislocation. It is surprising how seldom fractures involving the temporomandibular joint give rise to late symptoms.

Summary of the Treatment of Condylar Fractures.—

Extracapsular Fractures:—

1. Unilateral fracture or fracture dislocation of the condyle is treated by early movement with or without a very short period of immobilization during the painful immediate post-traumatic phase.

2. Bilateral fracture or fracture dislocation, where there is no anterior open bite, should be treated by early movements, with or without a short period of immobilization, as in (1).

3. Bilateral fractures or fracture dislocations, where there is an anterior open bite, present a more difficult problem. If the anterior open bite is not corrected considerable derangement of the occlusion results which may necessitate extraction of all the molar teeth in order to enable the patient to bite with the front teeth. Early treatment of such cases is necessary. Upper and lower cap splints are fitted and the occlusion is then gagged in the molar area with a small attachment to the lower splint or by inserting two or three thicknesses of gutta-percha sheeting between the opposing molar teeth after which the anterior open bite is reduced by powerful elastic traction between opposing hooks on the upper and lower splints in the incisor area.

This splintage distracts the ramus in the condylar region and the fixation is worn for about 6 weeks following closure of the anterior open bite. If the patient is edentulous the problem is less difficult, for the occlusal derangement can often be corrected prosthodontically.

Intracapsular Fractures.—The main complication arising in this type of fracture is that of bony ankylosis. To avoid this possibility early movement of the mandible is encouraged. Should this not prove successful a condylectomy may be necessary.

Fractures of the Condylar Region in Children.—The condylar growth centre may be damaged as a result of fracture in this region and this results in cessation of growth of the mandible on the affected side. Fortunately, many fractures of the condylar neck in children are greenstick in type, and therefore this disfiguring complication does not occur. Following all severe condylar fractures in children regular follow-up examinations are advisable until growth ceases, so that any failure of growth on one side of the mandible can be diagnosed. Walker (1957) investigated 50 cases demonstrating arrest in development of the mandibular condyle and found 14 out of 39 patients with unilateral ankylosis and 5 out of 11 with bilateral ankylosis; the condition resulted from trauma. The treatment of condylar fractures in children is similar to that adopted in adults, but it should be remembered that bony union occurs more rapidly in children and therefore very early movement of the joint should be encouraged. There is no indication for open reduction and transosseous wiring in the case of condylar fractures in children unless there is interference with mandibular movement (Rowe, 1969).

Cases of Persistent Deviation of the Bite.—As already stated, the bite tends to deviate towards the injured side and very occasionally this condition may persist. Treatment for such a deviation is by the use of a bite flange. This consists of a metal projection or flange which is attached to a lower splint on the opposite side to which the jaw is deviating. This flange engages an attachment on an upper splint and prevents the jaw deviating as the mouth is opened. There are two varieties of flange and these achieve active and passive training to correct the deviation.

The passive type of flange is constructed so that the flange on the lower splint engages a flat surface on an upper splint and the jaw is mechanically prevented from deviating. This device does little to train the musculature and when the apparatus is removed the patient usually lapses into the original pattern of jaw deviation. A more satisfactory treatment is the active type of training device which consists of a flange on a lower splint which clears the upper splint laterally on closing the mouth only if the patient makes a determined effort to prevent mandibular deviation. In this way the musculature is trained to avoid a deviation of the mandible and a permanent cure is achieved.

Chapter VII

DEFINITIVE TREATMENT OF FRACTURES OF THE RAMUS AND BODY OF THE MANDIBLE

The general principles of treatment of fractures of the mandible do not differ essentially from the treatment of fractures elsewhere in the body. The fragments are reduced into a good position and are then immobilized until such time as bony union occurs.

REDUCTION

Reduction is best effected under general anaesthesia, but occasionally it is possible to carry out reduction under local analgesia or while the patient is sedated with morphine gr. ¼ (15 mg.) or pethidine 100 mg. If there is minimal displacement the reduction can sometimes be effected without an anaesthetic. If teeth are present on the fragments gradual reduction of fractures can be carried out by elastic traction. To achieve this, cap splints or wires are fitted to the upper and lower teeth on the fragments and mandibular-maxillary elastic traction is applied between them. This method used to be popular, but it is not so effective as reduction under general anaesthesia. However, it is occasionally useful if the patient's general medical condition precludes the administration of a general anaesthetic.

Obviously if the teeth are restored to their normal position the bony fragments must also be correctly alined. Therefore, if teeth are present on the main fragments they may be used to effect the reduction, check the alinement of the fragments, and assist in the immobilization.

However, unless reduction is perfect the patient with a complete or almost complete dentition will have a derangement of the occlusion. Some latitude is possible if the patient is edentulous, for a less than perfect reduction of the fragments can be compensated when the dentures are constructed. Perfect reduction of the fracture is assumed if the teeth are restored to their normal alinement, but it is more difficult to judge the position of edentulous fragments unless an open reduction is carried out through either an extra-oral or an intra-oral incision.

TOOTH IN THE FRACTURE LINE

If the blood-supply to the pulp of a tooth is damaged as a result of a fracture of the mandible the pulp will, of course, die. Infection from the apex of such a tooth into the fracture line will result in greatly protracted healing of the fracture or even non-union. Therefore, if the viability of a tooth in the region of a fracture line is in doubt it should be extracted. It is possible, however, for a tooth alongside a fracture site not to be involved in the fracture and to have an unimpaired blood-supply to the pulp. In such a case careful examination of an intra-oral radiograph will reveal that the apex of the tooth is not involved and that there is a layer of intact bone over the periodontal membrane. There is no necessity to remove such a tooth. Indeed the extraction of the tooth, embedded as it is in sound bone, may require a degree of force which will disrupt the fracture line unnecessarily. For instance, a simple crack fracture could be converted into a severe displacement no matter how carefully the extraction was performed. The removal of the tooth either side of the fracture line is therefore only necessary if the blood-supply is impaired. It is impossible to be certain whether a tooth is involved in the fracture line from an examination of extra-oral radiographs, and careful intra-oral apical films studied in conjunction with occlusal films across the fracture line are necessary to evaluate the condition.

The radiographs should be assessed in conjunction with vitality tests on the teeth concerned. If a fracture passes in the vicinity of an unerupted lower third molar, it is best to leave the tooth in situ and carry out routine immobilization of the mandible unless the radiograph shows the tooth to be fractured. In most instances, a fracture which apparently passes through an unerupted tooth will heal satisfactorily provided it does not become infected. If the tooth is actually fractured, infection is more or less inevitable and it should be removed prior to immobilization of the jaw.

IMMOBILIZATION

Following accurate reduction of the fragments the mandible should be immobilized for a period of about 5 weeks if the patient is a normal healthy adult with an uninfected fracture.

Union of the fragments occurs more readily in children and immobilization for 3 weeks to a month is generally sufficient.

Old patients, and cases where the fracture has become infected, require a longer period of immobilization and 6 or 7 weeks is often necessary.

The main methods of immobilizing the mandible are:—
1. *Dental wiring.*
   This may be: (a) Direct or (b) Eyelet.
2. *Arch bars.*
3. *Silver–copper alloy cap splints.*
4. *Gunning-type splints.*
5. *Transosseous wiring.*
   This may be: (a) Upper border wiring or (b) Lower border wiring.
6. *External pin fixation.*
7. *Bone clamps.*
8. *Bone plating.*
9. *Transfixation with Steinmann pins or Kirschner wires.*

1. Dental Wiring.—Dental wiring is used when the patient has a complete or almost complete set of suitably shaped teeth. Opinions differ as to the type and gauge of wire used, but 0·35 mm. soft stainless-steel wire has been found effective. This wire requires stretching before use and should be stretched about 10 per cent. If this is not done the wires become slack after being in position a few days. Care should be taken not to over-stretch the wire as it will become work hardened and brittle.

Numerous techniques have been described for dental wiring, but two have been found very satisfactory. The most simple is direct wiring.

a. Direct Wiring.—The middle portion of a 6-inch (15-cm.) length of wire is twisted round a suitable tooth and then the free ends are twisted together to produce a 3- or 4-inch (7·5–10-cm.) length of 'plaited' wire.

Similar wires are attached to other teeth elsewhere in the upper and lower jaws and then after reduction of the fracture the plaited ends of wires in the upper and lower jaws are in turn twisted together (*Fig.* 15). For greater stability the wire surrounding each tooth can be applied in the form of a clove hitch. Thus suitable teeth in the upper and lower jaws are joined together by direct wires.

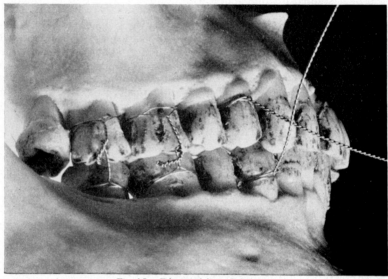

Fig. 15.—Direct wiring of the jaws.

This is a simple rapid method of immobilizing the jaws, especially if the special 'wire twister' is employed (*Fig.* 16), but it has the disadvantage that the mandibular–maxillary wires are connected to the teeth themselves. It is therefore difficult to release the mandibular–maxillary connexion without stripping off all the fixation. This disadvantage can be overcome by using interdental eyelet wiring.

b. Interdental Eyelet Wiring.—Eyelets are constructed by holding a 6-inch (15-cm.) length of wire by a pair of artery forceps at either end and giving the middle of the wire two turns round a piece of round bar $\frac{1}{8}$ in. or 3 mm. in diameter which is fixed in an upright position.

These eyelets are fitted between two teeth in the manner shown in the diagram and twisted tight (*Fig.* 17). Care must be taken to push the wire well down on the lingual and palatal aspect of the teeth before twisting the free ends tight, as the eyelet will tend to be displaced up the tooth and become loose. This can be done by pushing the wire down on the lingual and palatal aspect with an instrument such as a flat plastic.

About five eyelets are applied in the upper jaw and five in the lower jaw and then the eyelets are connected with tie wires passing through the eyelets from the upper to the lower jaw. To test whether a fracture is soundly united it is then possible to remove only the tie wires, and if a further period of immobilization is indicated new tie wires can be attached.

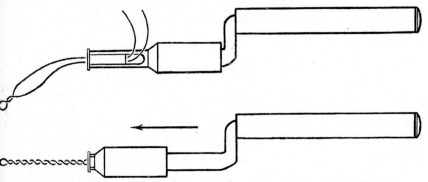

Fig. 16.—Diagram of a simple 'wire twister' for use in direct wiring. The wire is passed round a tooth and then the two free ends are inserted into the tube at the end of the instrument. They are directed up an inclined plane in the tube to emerge through a hole in its side. The free ends of wire are then immobilized by pushing forwards the loose circular sleeve, and on turning the handle of the instrument an even twisting of the wire is rapidly achieved.

The eyelets should be so positioned in the upper and the lower jaw that when the tie wires are threaded through them a cross-bracing effect is achieved. If the eyelets are placed immediately above each other some mobility of the mandible is possible. It should be remembered when working with wire that the wire is very sharp and very springy and could readily transfix a patient's eyeball if carelessly handled. Precautions must be taken to protect the eyes at all times and to achieve this object every free end of wire should have a pair of heavy artery forceps attached to it when it is not actually being manipulated.

When working under general anaesthesia the eyes should be closed and covered first with a layer of tulle gras and then a thick layer of polythene sponge. This in turn is covered with a sheet of thick rubber and outside this the anaesthetic harness holds all firmly in place.

After the eyelet wires are fixed the tie wires should be threaded through the eyelets so connecting the eyelets of the upper and lower jaw, but the tie wires are not twisted tight at this stage. Teeth which require extraction are removed at this time and before completing the mandibular–maxillary fixation the throat pack is removed, after which the fracture is reduced and the tie wire fixation is tightened.

It is important that the patient's normal pre-fracture occlusion is understood by the operator, for many patients have some abnormality of their occlusion and an attempt to achieve a theoretically correct occlusion in such cases may result in gross derangement of the bony fragments. Much information about the previous occlusion can be inferred from such evidence as facets on the teeth, but if the operator is in any doubt about the patient's correct occlusion, study models should be prepared before operation.

Tie wires should be tightened in the molar area, first on one side and then the other, so working round to the incisor area. It should be remembered that if the wires are tightened on one side first a cross-over bite is produced and if the anterior wires are tightened before the wires in the molar area a posterior open bite results. The wires may be twisted very tight on multi-rooted teeth, but some caution should be exercised with single-rooted teeth for they may be extracted as a result of force from twisting the tie wire over-tight.

It is best to twist the tie wires loosely together first and carry out the final tightening after the occlusion has been checked. Care must be taken to ensure that the tongue is not trapped between the cusps of the teeth.

After the interdental eyelet wiring is completed a finger should be run round the patient's mouth to ensure that no loose ends of wire have been left projecting which may ulcerate the soft tissue (*Fig.* 18). Interdental

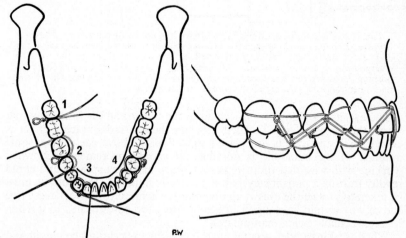

Fig. 17.—Diagram of the various stages in the insertion of an interdental eyelet wire.

Fig. 18.—A completed eyelet wiring showing how the eyelets are connected by the tie wires.

eyelet wiring is simple to apply and very effective in operation. Excellent reduction and immobilization is effected as the operator can see that the occlusion is perfectly restored. In practice more than half the total number of mandibular fractures of the so-called 'civilian type' can be treated in this fashion.

2. The Arch Bar.—Arch bars are used when the patient has an insufficient number of suitably shaped teeth to enable effective interdental eyelet wiring to be carried out. The method is very simple. The fracture is reduced and then the teeth on the main fragments are tied to a metal bar which has been bent to conform to the dental arch. Many varieties of prefabricated arch bar are available and the Winter-, Jelenko-, and Erich-type bars have all proved effective. These bars are supplied in suitable lengths and have hooks or other devices to assist in the maintenance of mandibular–maxillary fixation (*Fig.* 19). In the absence of such specialized bars a very effective arch bar can be constructed from $\frac{1}{8}$-in. (3-mm.) half-round German silver bar. Notches are cut on the bar with the edge of a file to prevent the mandibular–maxillary tie wires from slipping.

Arch bars should be cut to the required length and bent to the correct shape before starting the operation. As the mandibular fragments are displaced owing to the fracture the bar is bent so that it fits around the upper arch. In practice it has been found that such a bar is quite satisfactory when applied to the lower arch as extreme accuracy is not required. When it is impossible to adapt the bar to the patient's upper teeth any lower plaster model of approximately the correct size can be used or the bar can be bent to fit another patient of approximately the same size of arch. To facilitate the bending of the German silver bar, it should be annealed by heating it red-hot and then allowing it to cool.

Faced for the first time with the problem of attaching an arch bar to a number of teeth by twisting lengths of 0·35-mm. soft stainless-steel wire around the teeth and over the bar, any operator would rapidly find a satisfactory solution. In fact, every operator has his own ideal method of achieving this result.

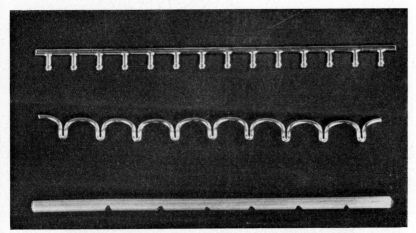

Fig. 19.—From above downwards, two useful forms of prefabricated arch bar, manufactured by Krupp, together with a length of half round German silver bar with notches cut into it with a file.

An elementary method is to twist the middle portion of 6-in, (15-cm.) lengths of wire around suitable teeth in the form of a clove hitch. When an adequate number of teeth has been ringed in this way the fracture is reduced and the arch bar laid alongside the teeth, the two free ends of the wire attached to the teeth passing above and below the bar in every case. The two free ends of 0·35-mm. wire are then twisted tightly together over the bar (*Fig.* 20). The free end of the twisted wire is then tucked into a position where it will not irritate the tissues.

Arch bars are a very effective method of fixation and are used when facilities for such techniques as cap splints are either not available or cannot be completed in time. Most fractures of the mandible can be effectively treated in this fashion if teeth are present on the main fragments (*Figs.* 21, 22).

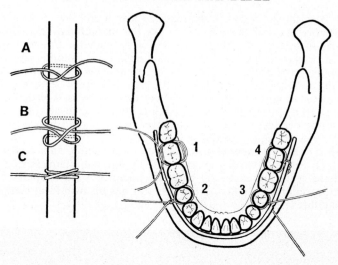

P.W

Fig. 20.—A method of attaching an arch bar to the teeth. The wire is passed round a tooth in the form of a clove hitch and then the free ends are threaded above and below the arch bar and twisted together. A, B, and C show the stages in the tying of a clove-hitch knot.

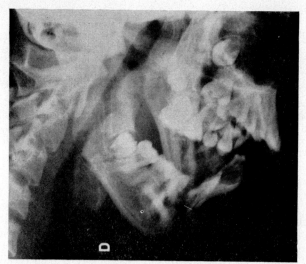

Fig. 21.—Radiograph of a severe mandibular fracture.

3. Cap Splints.—This method is used when few teeth are available on the main fragments and such splinting produces a very rigid fixation even when only one tooth is present on a fragment. The laboratory technique for the construction of splints cannot be dealt with adequately in a book of this nature and only practical aspects in the application of such splints will be considered. So far as the actual construction of cap splints is concerned it is sufficient to say that the technique is complicated and requires the services of skilled laboratory technicians. It is therefore more costly and not readily available outside specially equipped maxillofacial centres. Operators who do not possess such facilities will therefore prefer to use other cheaper and more readily available methods for treating their fractures. The use of cap splints has also been criticized on the grounds that their construction is a lengthy process and that it is impossible to achieve a perfect occlusion in the treated case owing to the thickness of splint metal over the crowns of the teeth. However, an efficient mechanical laboratory can construct cap splints in from 6 to 8 hours and if they are correctly made there should be an almost perfect restoration of the occlusion. This is achieved by fitting the completed splints on models in an articulator and grinding the bite between the opposing splints into correct occlusion.

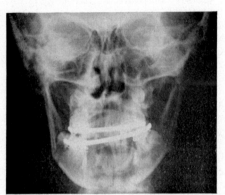
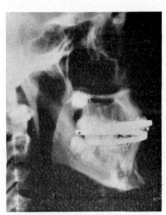

Figs. 22.—Radiographs of injury shown in *Fig.* 21 following reduction and immobilization with arch bars.

Impression Technique.—Before taking an impression the mouth and teeth must be cleaned and dried blood, etc., removed from the tooth surfaces.

Impressions are required of the tooth surfaces only and therefore a lower impression tray can be used in the upper jaw. Patients with a fractured mandible find it painful to open the mouth fully and the use of a lower tray is more comfortable for them. Trays are cut down to about half the normal depth and this again facilitates their manipulation in the mouth. Teeth on individual fragments must have their own individual impression tray, for an overall impression is seldom practical when the fragments are displaced. Some soft impression material, such as one of the hydrocolloids (Zelex, etc.), causes the patient least discomfort and produces an accurate impression. The splints can therefore be constructed on an accurate model, but care must be taken to fill in undercuts before making the splint or it will be impossible to fit the splint on the teeth.

Some operators prefer composition impression material. This is more uncomfortable for the patient as very firm pressure is required on the mobile fragments. Such impression material drags, as it is removed, and the impression is less accurate. However, the drag has the advantage that undercuts do not require filling out on the model and the splint can be constructed directly to the model.

Workroom Instructions.—The operator should examine the model when it is cast and give careful instructions to the technician concerning the construction of the splint. It is wise to mark with an indelible pencil the position of locking plates, hooks, etc., and place a cross on the teeth which are to be extracted. Such teeth must, of course, be left out of the splint.

Fitting the Splint.—The completed splints should be tried on the teeth. Every tooth cusp on the splint must be provided with a small vent to allow excess cement to escape and while the splint is in position on the teeth a probe may be passed down these holes to ensure that the cusp is immediately beneath the metal and that the splint fits accurately.

The splint and teeth are then dried and kept free of saliva by the use of swabs either side of the arch. The ends of the swabs are left hanging out of the mouth so that they can be rapidly removed when the splint is inserted into the mouth at the time of cementing. The under-surface of the splint is then coated with black Ames copper cement mixed fairly thinly, the swabs are removed, and the splint pressed into position on the teeth. To ensure that it is accurately adapted to the cusps a probe is again passed through the vents on the surface to confirm that the tooth cusp is immediately beneath the splint. To prevent cement entering screw holes in the locking plates or beneath hooks all these areas should be filled with wax before cementing. When the cement has hardened, all excess cement is removed with a scaler. The wax under the hooks is removed at this time but wax in the screw holes is left until the localization as they may otherwise become filled with blood or food debris, etc.

Ames copper cement is very effective but it is, of course, dirty and some operators prefer to use a quick-setting acrylic for this purpose. Patients occasionally experience some pain in the teeth after the splint has been cemented with Ames copper cement. This passes off in about 6 hours, and can be relieved with a mild analgesic such as 2 tabs. codeine co.

Reduction of Fracture.—The fracture is reduced manually or by gradual elastic traction from rubber bands between hooks on the upper and lower splint. In either instance the fracture is temporarily immobilized by mandibular–maxillary elastic traction and then the various sections of the lower splints are joined by constructing a locking bar (*Figs.* 23, 24). The various portions of splint must, of course, be immobilized while localization proceeds.

Localization.—Localization is carried out with locking plates and connecting bars. Two main types of locking plate are in use: (1) The Fickling type oval locking plate; (2) The brass locking plate originally introduced by Macleod and Shepherd in 1941.

The Fickling locking plate has the advantage that it is more easily applied when considerable lengths of bar are required, for the pin in the brass-type locking plate tends to interfere with adaptation of the locking plates in such cases.

The risk of local electrolytic action is more likely when the brass locking plate is used, but ulceration of the opposing soft tissues can be prevented by coating the plate with sticky wax.

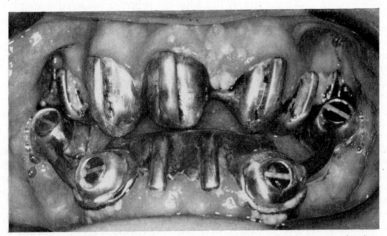

Fig. 23.—Silver-copper alloy cap splints with locking plates and connecting bars used in the treatment of a bilateral fracture of the body of the mandible. The mandibular–maxillary fixation with rubber bands between the hooks has been removed in order to demonstrate the locking plates and connecting bars more clearly.

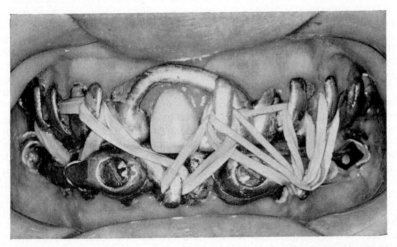

Fig. 24.—If there is only a single tooth on each posterior fragment it is occasionally difficult to retain such small cap splints on these teeth. A satisfactory fixation can be achieved in such cases by soldering an arch bar to a locking plate on the anterior fragment and wiring the posterior tooth directly to the arch bar. The upper splint should be thickened to compensate for the fact that the lower posterior tooth has no covering of splint metal. This will ensure that the bite is correct when treatment is completed.

Locking plates are fitted to the locking plate bases with screws and for ease of manipulation during localization the 6.BA screws have a handle attached to them. On the surface of each locking plate, distal to the neighbouring locking plate of the adjacent splint, is soldered a length of No. 8 wire and this is bent over a similar wire attached to the neighbouring locking plate. It is important that these wires do not touch each other, or tension between the two wires will spring the two locking plates into an incorrect position when their screws are removed. Plaster-of-Paris is then run over the two free ends of wire and an accelerator in the water ensures a rapid set of plaster. It is then possible to remove the screws from the locking plates and by holding the plaster, the locking plates are lifted gently clear of the splints. The plaster and wire ensure that the plates are held in exactly the same position as they occupied on the splints.

The locking plates are then taken to the mechanical laboratory and a suitable length of ⅛-in. (3-mm.) half-round German silver bar is soldered between them. The original round wire used for localization is cut off the locking plates and the completed connecting bar and locking plates are finally attached to the splints with ordinary 6.BA screws. In this fashion the various splints cemented to teeth in the main fragments are connected together and the mandibular fractures are immobilized (*Figs.* 25–28). Mandibular–maxillary fixation is effected by elastic traction between the hooks on the upper and lower splints. Fixation with elastic bands allows a very slight movement should the patient try to yawn or grind the teeth at night, and this reduces the force on the copper cement seal. Rigid mandibular–maxillary fixation with connecting bars from upper to lower locking plates or the use of wire between the hooks means that the thin layer of cement is subjected to continuous direct strain and may crack. The splint would then become detached.

Local electrolytic action may occur on the German silver bar producing an ulcer on the overlying soft tissues. This ulcer will heal in about a week when the bar becomes coated with an oxide film, but these painful ulcers are best prevented by coating the bar with sticky wax at the time it is fitted.

4. Modified Gunning-type Splints.—This technique is used when the patient is edentulous in one or both jaws. If the patient is completely edentulous immobilization is carried out by attaching modified Gunning-type splints to the upper jaw by peralveolar wires and to the lower jaw by circumferential wires, after which mandibular–maxillary fixation is effected by connecting the two splints with elastic bands. When the patient is edentulous in one jaw mandibular–maxillary fixation is carried out by attaching the Gunning splints to whatever type of splinting is present in the opposing jaw.

Gunning splints take the form of a denture with bite-blocks in place of molar teeth and a space in the incisor area to facilitate feeding. If the correct vertical dimensions of the bite are known some interdigitating locking device is carved on the occlusal surface of the bite-blocks in the molar region. If the correct bite is not known a trough filled with black gutta percha is cut in the occlusal surface of one bite-block and the opposing block is shaped to fit into this trough (*Figs.* 29, 30). At operation the gutta percha is softened and the approximate bite obtained by pressing one splint into the gutta percha in the trough of the opposing splint.

The fitting surface of the splints is lined with black gutta percha to prevent the hard acrylic from chafing the alveolar ridges. The splints may be constructed on models made from impressions taken of the patient's mouth, but as the mandible is fractured it is often impossible to obtain an accurate lower impression.

Localization Technique

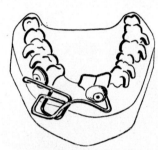

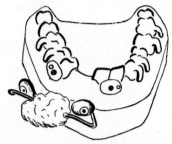

Fig. 25.—Locking plates in position with wire soldered to their outer aspects. These wires are bent over each other, taking care that they do not touch. The plates are then held in position with mounted screws which are not shown on the diagram.

Fig. 26.—Plaster-of-Paris is run over the free ends of the wires and when this is set the locking plates are held in the position they occupy on the splints.

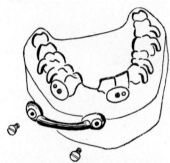

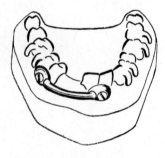

Fig. 27.—A length of ⅛-in. (3-mm.) half-round German silver bar is soldered between the inner borders of the opposing locking plates. The wires previously attached to their outer aspects have been cut off.

Fig. 28.—Locking plates and connecting bars screwed into position on the splints.

Most edentulous patients possess dentures and plaster models can be cast using their fitting surfaces as an impression. If the patient's dentures were broken at the time of the accident it is well worth while repairing them so that they can be used to provide an accurate pre-accident model of the lower ridge from which splints can be constructed.

Satisfactory Gunning-type splints can be made using the patient's dentures, if they are available. To do this the fitting surface of the dentures is greased with petroleum jelly after which they are pressed on to a mound of wet plaster-of-Paris, so casting models of the patient's alveolus. The entire fitting surface of the dentures is then drilled away to the depth of about ⅛ in. (3 mm.) using a large rosehead bur in a dental engine. A

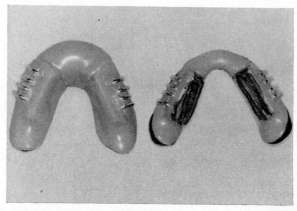

Fig. 29.—Gunning-type splints. The lower splint on the right has a trough on its upper surface filled with gutta percha into which the upper splint fits. This enables the vertical dimension of the bite to be adjusted.

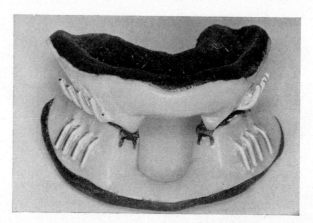

Fig. 30.—Upper and lower Gunning-type splints showing fitting surface of splints lined with gutta percha.

sheet of gutta percha is heated and placed on the undersurface of the dentures which are then pressed down on to the plaster-of-Paris models. Thus the dentures are re-lined with black gutta percha. The anterior teeth of the dentures are removed to provide a space for feeding, hooks are fitted to the sides of the upper and lower denture for use in mandibular–maxillary fixation and grooves are cut in the upper and lower canine region to contain the peralveolar and circumferential wires.

At operation the upper splint is fixed to the alveolus by using an awl to pass an 0·5-mm. soft stainless-steel wire through the alveolus high up in the canine area on each side and tying the two free ends over the upper Gunning-type splint.

Circumferential wires are passed round the mandible in the canine region with the aid of needles, awls, or cannulae. The easiest methods are

Professor Obwegeser's Technique for Circumferential Wiring

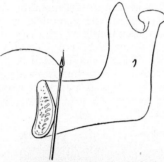

Fig. 31.—An awl is pushed through the skin beneath the chin and up into the mouth on the lingual side of the mandible. A length of 0·5-mm. soft stainless-steel wire is threaded into its tip.

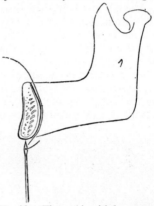

Fig. 32.—The awl is withdrawn to the lower border of the mandible.

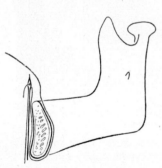

Fig. 33.—Keeping the awl close to the bone it is passed round the lower border and then pushed up into the buccal sulcus.

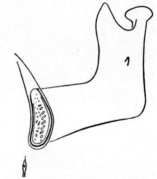

Fig. 34.—The wire is detached from the tip of the awl and the instrument is then withdrawn from the tissues through the external wound.

either to thread a large Hagedorn curved cutting needle with 0·5-mm. soft stainless-steel wire and pass it with the concavity outwards down the lingual side of the mandible and out under the jaw. The needle is then inserted through the exit hole and passed again with the concavity outwards up the buccal side of the mandible. Each end of the wire is then held in a pair of Spencer Wells forceps and with a sawing motion the circumferential wire cuts through the overlying soft tissues until it reaches the bone. Each circumferential wire is then tied over the lower Gunning splint. 'Sawing' the stainless-steel wire against the lower border of the mandible causes the length of the wire in contact with the bone to become work hardened. It is therefore necessary to use an adequate length of wire to enable the sawing action to be accomplished at one end and when the wire is resting against the bone it is then pulled round so that a fresh length of wire is tied over the lower Gunning splint.

Probably the easiest and best method is Professor Obwegeser's technique. A small awl is pushed through the skin beneath the mandible and brought out in the mouth on the lingual side of the mandible, in the canine area. It is threaded with the wire and then gently withdrawn to the lower border of the mandible, but not out through the skin. The tip of the awl is guided round the lower border of the mandible and is then pushed up into the buccal sulcus where the wire is detached from the awl and the instrument is withdrawn from the original puncture wound beneath the chin. As the wire is already against the lower border it is unnecessary to saw through the soft tissues (*Figs*. 31–34).

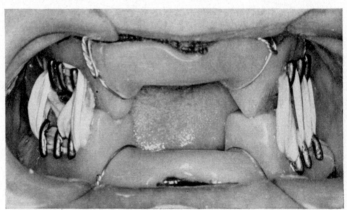

Fig. 35.—Gunning-type splints, showing circumferential and per-alveolar wires in position. Mandibular–maxillary fixation is effected with elastic bands between the upper and lower hooks.

When the Gunning-type splints are fixed to both upper and lower jaws they are connected with elastic bands between the upper and lower hooks to achieve mandibular–maxillary fixation (*Fig*. 35).

When treatment is completed, the peralveolar and circumferential wires are removed quite simply by cutting one end and pulling the wire through. An anaesthetic is not required, but as infection may be carried deep into the tissues the sulcus in the region of the wire should be carefully cleaned with antiseptic lotion and the patient should be given an antibiotic as a prophylactic measure.

5. Transosseous Wiring.—Transosseous wiring is an extremely effective method of immobilizing a fracture of the mandible. Holes are drilled in the bone ends on either side of the fracture line and after reduction of the fracture a 0·5-mm. soft stainless-steel wire is passed through the holes and across the fracture, after which the free ends are twisted tight, cut off short, and the twisted end tucked into the nearest drill hole. Transosseous wiring is especially useful in the treatment of edentulous mandibular fractures or for the control of the edentulous posterior fragment. It can be

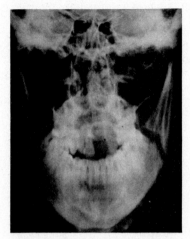 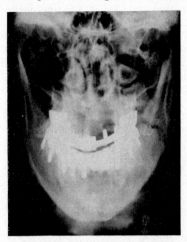

Fig. 36.—Radiograph of fracture at angle of mandible.

Fig. 37.—Radiograph of upper border transosseous wire in position in fracture shown in Fig. 36.

carried out at the lower border of the mandible through an extra-oral surgical approach or at the upper border from an intra-oral incision.

It is important that the fracture is not infected if a transosseous wire

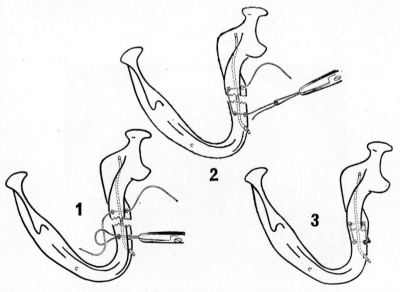

Fig. 38—Technique for inserting transosseous wires.

is to be inserted owing to the risk of necrosis of the bone ends. At one time it was considered inadvisable to insert a lower border wire if the fracture was compound into the mouth because of the risk of infection, but with the use of suitable antibiotics, such as tetracycline, the risk is negligible.

Upper border wiring is effected through an intra-oral incision along the crest of the alveolus, and it is often sufficient for the alveolus alone to be drilled and wired after which the wound is carefully sutured (*Figs.* 36–38). If an upper border wire becomes infected it can be removed quite easily, but an infected lower border wire is more difficult to reach.

It is technically possible to fit a lower border wire from an intra-oral incision and so avoid an external scar. A problem arises with lower border wiring of a bilateral fracture through the body of the mandible, for

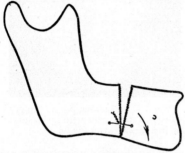

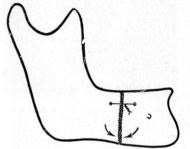

Fig. 39.—Diagram of lower border wire showing that muscular pull on the anterior fragment tends to make the upper end of the fracture line gape. This most commonly occurs in bilateral fractures and it can, to a certain extent, be overcome by using a figure-of-eight-type wiring at the lower border.

Fig. 40.—An upper border wire showing that the pull of the muscles on the anterior fragment tends to impact the ends and prevent the displacement illustrated in *Fig.* 39.

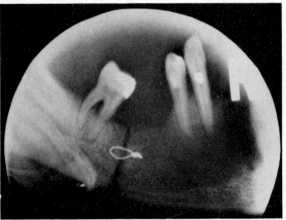

Fig. 41.—Radiograph showing transosseous wire inserted above mandibular canal as illustrated in *Fig.* 40.

owing to muscular pull in the region of the chin the upper end of the fracture has a tendency to gape. This can be overcome to a certain extent by using a figure-of-eight type of wiring at the lower border or combining the transosseous wiring with some other type of fixation such as Gunning-type splints. This mandibular–maxillary fixation will ensure that the anterior fragment does not sag. The use of upper border wires through the mandible immediately below the level of the alveolar bone avoids the tendency of the upper part of the fracture to gape, for under these circum-stances the pull of the muscles in the mental region only tends to impact the bone ends together (*Figs.* 39–41).

Transosseous wiring has the advantage that minimal specialized equipment is required apart from 0·5-mm. soft stainless-steel wire, and this method can be used to treat all mandibular fractures which cannot be satisfactorily treated with eyelet or arch wiring. It is, of course, unnecessary to remove the transosseous wire at the conclusion of treatment. Transosseous wiring must not be used if the fracture is infected for the presence of the metallic 'foreign body' may cause bone necrosis.

6. Extra-oral Pin Fixation.—Extra-oral pin fixation is seldom required for the treatment of civilian-type fractures of the mandible, The technique consists of inserting into each bone fragment a pair of $\frac{1}{8}$-in. (3-mm.) stainless-steel pins which diverge from each other, but are connected by a cross-bar which is attached to each pin by a joint. Although the pins have sharp points they should not be drilled into the bone for fear of splitting it. Instead a hole should be drilled with a twist drill of slightly smaller diameter and then the pin is inserted into this hole. The principle is similar to that employed by a cabinet maker when inserting wood screws so as to avoid splitting the wood. From the centre of the cross-bar a joint secures a short length of $\frac{1}{8}$-in. (3-mm.) stainless-steel rod and to the end of this rod a universal joint is attached. The fracture is reduced and then the various pairs of pins are connected by fixing $\frac{1}{8}$-in. (3-mm.) stainless-steel rod between the various universal joints.

Pin fixation is by no means rigid and supplementary mandibular–maxillary fixation is often required. Electrolytic action can occur with pin fixation and this may produce ring sequestra in the bone and ulceration of the skin where the pin is inserted. As the pins project from the patient's jaw they may easily be inadvertently traumatized. Patients with this form of fixation are of necessity somewhat conspicuous and it is therefore usually necessary for them to remain in hospital throughout the period of fixation.

There are few occasions when the fracture could not be immobilized more effectively by transosseous wiring, but if the fracture line is infected pin fixation is occasionally a helpful means of effecting immobilization.

7. Bone Clamps.—Another form of external fixation for mandibular fractures is the use of bone clamps. Instead of pins drilled into the bone the fragments are grasped by clamps inserted from an external approach. The protruding ends of the clamps are joined by connecting bars and universal joints in a similar manner to that employed with the external pin fixation. The Brenthurst clamp is the best known and most effective clamp of this nature and a similar apparatus has been described by Professor Rudko, of Moscow.

Bone clamps have the same advantages and disadvantages already mentioned in the discussion of external pin fixation.

8. Bone Plating.—The main advantage of bone plating for the treatment of mandibular fractures is that it provides an extremely rigid fixation, and it is therefore unnecessary to immobilize the mandible. This enables the patient to enjoy a normal diet and there is, of course, a reduced period of treatment. The special clinical advantages are in those cases of mandibular fracture where early mobilization of the temporomandibular joint is

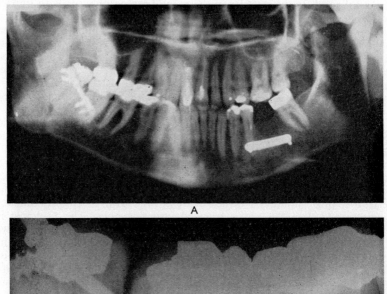

A

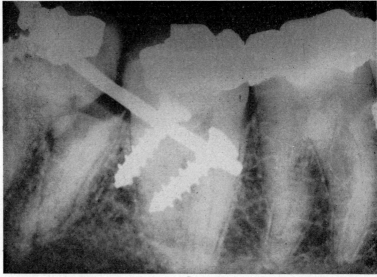

B

Fig. 42.—**A**, Orthopantomogram showing bilateral fracture of the mandible which has been treated with bone plates which have been inserted through an intra-oral approach. Insertion of one of the screws has fractured the anterior root of the $\overline{5|}$ and this has caused non-union on that side. **B**, Periapical film showing the fractured root.

required in order to prevent possible ankylosis. It is also advantageous not having to rely on specialized maxillofacial laboratory help in the treatment of the fracture. However, the patient requires a general anaesthetic, and as the plates are inserted from an external approach a residual scar remains on the face at the conclusion of treatment. Bone plates may be inserted from an intra-oral approach but this increases the risk of infection and if teeth are present in the vicinity of the plate there is the risk of the screws damaging the roots of the teeth (*Fig.* 42). Bone plates must never be used if the fracture line is infected owing to the risk of severe bone necrosis.

The bone plates are vitallium metacarpal bone plates 1 in. or $\frac{3}{4}$ in. (2·5 cm. or 1·875 cm.) in length, and they should have four holes. Vitallium screws are used and these must be worked with a special vitallium screwdriver. Battersby (1967) reported a series of 350 fractures treated by this method between 1953 and 1963 and he analysed 60 of these. Union occurred in all cases, but 24 had residual paraesthesia of the lip, 6 had bad scars, in 6 cases the wound discharged pus, and the plate had to be removed in 1 case.

Compression Bone Plates.—Even though a mandibular fracture is immobilized with a bone plate at the lower border, there is still a tendency for the fracture line to distract at its upper end due to muscular pull when the mouth is opened and this may lead to a distorted occlusion. In addition, fixation of a plate on one side of the mandible leads to widening of the fracture on the opposite side (Spiessl, 1972).

In order to overcome these and other problems the compression bone plate has been developed. This is a four-screw plate and the two centre holes are pear-shaped and when in use they have their widest diameter facing towards the fracture line. The screws are inserted in the narrow part of the hole and only when they are tightened does the head of the screw come to rest in the widest diameter of the hole which is counter sunk to receive it. Tightening of the two central screws either side of the fracture line therefore compresses the bone ends together, after which the two outer screws are inserted to stabilize the plate. Unfortunately the use of a compression bone plate at the lower border tends to open the fracture line at its upper end even more widely than when the conventional bone plate is used and to overcome this problem some routine intra-oral fixation is necessary to secure good occlusion. This may take the form of interdental eyelet wiring or the use of an arch bar and this fixation is further stabilized with acrylic. It is necessary to do this so that while manipulating the fragments during operation good occlusion is guaranteed.

After surgery to fix the compression plates this inter-maxillary fixation is removed. A very exact and meticulous technique has been developed by Spiessl (1972).

An extra-oral approach is made to the fracture line. The bone fragments are manipulated and immobilized with the help of special forceps. First two 10-mm. screws are inserted to about half their depth into the inferior surface of the lower border of the mandible on either side and about 1 cm. from the fracture line. The ends of the special forceps fit over the protruding heads of these screws and after the fragments have been manipulated into satisfactory apposition the blades of the forceps are clamped together so holding the fragments quite rigid.

The bone plate should have a slight bend with the concavity away from the bone surface so that when the plate is screwed firmly into place there is no tendency for the fracture line to gape on its lingual aspect. When the two central screws of the plate are in place the special clamp is removed and the screws in the inferior border are removed. The two outer screws are then inserted in the plate and the wound is closed.

This entire process is lengthy especially when an extra-oral approach is made bilaterally and it should be remembered that routine intra-oral fixation has to be in place before the extra-oral operation is begun. The advantage of not having inter-maxillary fixation at the conclusion of the operation is not as complete as might be expected for after a bilateral external approach to the mandible the patient is not able to eat with any degree of comfort for about three weeks. This is no great advantage over the normal 5-week period of immobilization with conventional methods of fixation. There are various complications of compression bone plates, the most important being metal fatigue fracture of the plate, necrosis of the bone ends, fracture of the small fragments of bone ends as the screws are inserted etc., but the most worrying possibility is undoubtedly the risk of infection at the fracture site with bone necrosis and extrusion of all the metallic foreign bodies. It would certainly be most inadvisable to insert any form of bone plating if there is any risk of the fracture site being infected.

9. Transfixation.—Fixation of fractures in the symphyseal region can be effected by reducing the fracture and then transfixing them by drilling a Steinmann pin or Kirschner wire through the fragments. The technique is most applicable and effective in cases which can, however, be immobilized more easily by any of the other techniques already described. The method was described by Des Prez and Kiehn (1959), Brown and McDowell (1942), and Dingman and Natvig (1964), who refer to it as the 'shish kebab' method.

Selection of an Immobilization Technique.—It is a comparatively simple matter to select the most suitable method of immobilization for any particular case of mandibular fracture. After a careful general medical examination of the patient and local clinical examination of the fracture, such factors as the general state of the patient, presence of teeth on main fragments, etc., will suggest the most obvious line of treatment. If teeth are present dental wiring, direct or eyelet, arch wiring, or cap splints may be used according to the number and distribution of the teeth.

Fractures in edentulous patients or edentulous fragments may be controlled by Gunning-type splints, transosseous wiring at the upper or lower border, by pin fixation, bone plating, or by transfixation techniques with Steinmann pins or Kirschner wires.

Often more than one technique would be suitable. For instance, cap splints can be used in all cases where teeth are present on the main fragments, even when there is a complete dentition.

It is also obvious that more than one immobilization technique may be necessary in treating a particular fracture.

The majority of mandibular fractures can be successfully treated with eyelet or arch wiring, Gunning-type splints, and transosseous wiring, and the other methods are only occasionally required.

CHAPTER VIII

POSTOPERATIVE CARE

THE postoperative care of a patient with a fracture of the mandible may be divided into three phases:—
1. The immediate postoperative phase when the patient is recovering from the general anaesthetic.
2. The intermediate phase during which time the mandibular–maxillary fixation is in position.
3. The late postoperative phase which includes the removal of the mandibular–maxillary fixation, bite rehabilitation, mobilization of the temporomandibular joints, and long term follow-up.

1. THE IMMEDIATE POSTOPERATIVE PHASE

Most maxillofacial units have a special recovery ward or intensive care unit to which patients are transferred from the operating theatre and there they are kept under skilled nursing supervision until they are fully recovered from the anaesthetic and fit to be transferred back to their ward. In the absence of such facilities an experienced nurse should remain with the patient until recovery is complete.

If mandibular–maxillary fixation has been carried out it is prudent to have available at the patient's bedside instruments such as scissors, wire cutters, screwdrivers, etc., so that the fixation could be removed in an emergency. It is also essential that good lighting is provided and that accessory lighting is available in case of a power failure. Patients should be returned from the theatre with a nasopharyngeal airway in position and this should be left in situ until the patient recovers consciousness. Control of the tongue in the unconscious patient can be effected if the surgeon inserts a tongue suture at the end of operation. The suture is passed using a large cutting needle which is inserted transversely into the back of the dorsum of the tongue after which a pair of haemostats are attached to the free ends of the suture. Traction on this suture will pull the tongue forwards. A gap can usually be found through the mandibular–maxillary fixation to enable the suture to protrude from the mouth. When no longer required one end of the suture is cut and the other end pulled through.

Patients should be nursed lying on their sides during recovery to enable any saliva or oozing blood to escape through the fixation. An efficient suction apparatus must be at the patient's bedside and to the sucker nozzle a length of $\frac{1}{8}$-in. (3-mm.) rubber or polythene tubing is attached. This enables the nurse to pass the tube down the nasopharyngeal airway or the nares to suck out the nasopharynx. The rubber or polythene suction tube can also be passed along the buccal sulcus to keep this area free of secretions.

If the patient is correctly prepared for operation by withholding food for 4 hours, postoperative vomiting presents no problem. If the patient should vomit the material is watery and will pass easily through the fixation. Skilled anaesthesia will reduce the incidence of postoperative vomiting to negligible proportions.

An occasional problem arises when a fracture patient requires an operation shortly after admission and the anaesthetist is uncertain whether the patient's stomach contains food. In these circumstances it is prudent to pass a stomach tube and evacuate the stomach contents before anaesthetizing the patient.

If external pin fixation has been used care must be taken if the patient is restless during recovery to avoid damage to the fixation apparatus and injury to the nursing staff.

2. Intermediate Postoperative Phase

General Supervision.—Patients who have sustained a maxillofacial injury and are hospitalized should be carefully examined at both a morning and evening ward round. The fixation must be checked to see that the splints have not become loose and the fracture site should be examined to ensure that satisfactory progress is being maintained. An adequately reduced and immobilized fracture is relatively painless and the post-traumatic oedema rapidly subsides. Any increase in swelling over the fracture site or the onset of pain with increasing tenderness on palpation over the site of injury and/or a rise in body temperature indicates some adverse development which requires immediate attention.

Posture.—Patients with a fracture of the mandible find it more comfortable if they are in the sitting position with the chin well forward and providing there is no contra-indication to this posture such as a fractured vertebra the conscious patient should be nursed in this position. The comatose or stuperose patient is best nursed lying on the side so that saliva and blood can dribble out of the mouth.

Sedation.—If the fracture has been adequately reduced and effectively immobilized, the patient will experience very little pain and postoperative analgesics are seldom indicated and should not be administered routinely.

It should be remembered that morphia in particular depresses the respiratory centre and cough reflex. If given intra-muscularly when the patient is shocked it remains where it is deposited and when the circulation improves it is rapidly absorbed and if more than one dose has been administered it may then give rise to morphine poisoning. The use of powerful analgesics such as morphine may mask a deteriorating level of consciousness, and it also masks severe pain of such conditions as peritonitis and causes a miosis which obscures the important physical sign of dilatation of the pupil in cerebral haemorrhage. Its use pre- and immediately postoperatively is contra-indicated in mandibular fracture cases. For the cerebrally irritated patient 5–8 ml. of paraldehyde intra-muscularly is safe and efficient, but it should be remembered that restlessness in a semi-conscious patient may be due to an obstructed airway or an overfull bladder.

Prevention of Infection.—To prevent the fracture haematoma becoming infected the patient should be given an antibiotic such as 1 mega unit of penicillin daily for 4 days. It is much easier to prevent infection of the fracture site than to cure an established infection.

Oral Hygiene.—Effective oral hygiene also plays an important part in the prevention of infection of the fracture line. The conscious patient is given hot normal saline mouthwashes following every meal and patients whose fractures are immobilized by any of the wiring techniques (direct, eyelet, or arch) or by silver–copper alloy cap splints can keep the fixation clean by using a toothbrush in the usual manner.

If the patient is too ill to cooperate in these simple measures to promote oral hygiene the mouth must be cleaned by the nursing staff after every meal using normal saline solution which is squirted into the mouth with a Higginson syringe. Care must be taken not to direct the stream of fluid down the site of any compounded fractures, so introducing infection. For the same reason, hydrogen peroxide mouthwashes should not be used as the oxygen bubbles may carry infected debris into fractures which are compounded into the mouth. Cap splints can be cleaned with a 1–4 per cent sodium bicarbonate solution on cotton-wool swabs held in forceps. Rubber bands may become soiled with food and should be changed when this occurs. Following the mouth toilet the lips should be smeared with petroleum jelly to prevent them becoming dry and sticking together.

Immediately following operation the saliva tends to become thick and ropey and this condition continues for a period of about 24 hours. There is also a tendency for the lips to stick together at this time. If the patient has a complete set of teeth which have been wired together, or if there are full upper and lower cap splints, the ropey saliva tends to occlude the interstices in the fixation and hinder oral respiration. The lips sticking together has, of course, a similar effect. The patient can be made very much more comfortable during this period if the mouth is cleaned at regular intervals with moist saline swabs and the lips are liberally lubricated with petroleum jelly.

Feeding.—The problem of providing a patient suffering from a maxillo-facial injury with adequate nutrition varies according to whether the subject is conscious and cooperative or is uncooperative due to a low level of consciousness or to cerebral irritation.

The Conscious Cooperative Patient.—The majority of patients with a fractured mandible can be fed by mouth even though their jaws are immobilized. Depending upon the size of the gaps in their fixation they can eat a semi-solid or a liquid diet. The normal diet is minced and then passed through a wire sieve of 16 meshes to the inch (every 2·5 cm.) and mixed with soup. An electric food mixer with a liquidizer attachment is invaluable for this purpose. The resultant fluid is sucked through the fixation into the mouth. A feeding cup with a spout to which an 8-in. (20-cm.) length of rubber tubing is attached enables patients to feed themselves by passing the end of the rubber tubing through a gap in the fixation or round the back of the lower teeth in the retro-molar fossa region. Flexible drinking straws such as Flex-straw (Hygienic Drinking Straws Co. Ltd., Bristol) are also very helpful to enable a patient in bed to drink from a vessel.

Liquid meals should be served at 2-hourly intervals, for too much fluid at one sitting can be nauseating.

The diet is supplemented with vitamins and protein preparations such as Complan. A diet of 2000–2500 calories is adequate to maintain nutritional equilibrium. The dietitian should endeavour to maintain the patient's interest in the diet by the use of flavouring agents and the food should be presented in as attractive a manner as possible. If the patient cannot swallow, a transnasal gastric tube is passed and a high calorie continuous drip feed is given (*Fig*. 43).

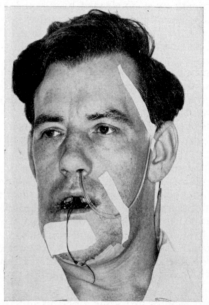

Fig. 43.—A Portex transnasal gastric tube in a patient who was unable to swallow. A tongue suture has been inserted as a precautionary measure.

The Unconscious or Uncooperative Patient.—

Fluid Balance.—A fluid balance chart should be kept for all patients suffering from maxillofacial injuries until such time as the clinician in charge of the case is satisfied that an adequate fluid intake is being voluntarily ingested by the patient.

The normal daily intake of water is about 3000 ml. and the output is made up of 1500 ml. of insensible loss by evaporation from the skin, sweating, etc., and 1500 ml. of urine.

It should be remembered that all forms of trauma and operations provoke a complex metabolic disturbance which varies directly with the magnitude and duration of the trauma or operation. This consists essentially of an inability to excrete water and salt with an increased metabolism and excretion of potassium and nitrogen. The impairment of water excretion lasts 24–36 hours and is characterized by low output of urine of high specific gravity. The impairment of secretion of sodium lasts 4–6 days, and after 24 hours there is marked lowering of sodium and chlorine in the urine. There is an increased excretion of potassium which lasts 24–48 hours due to mobilization and excretion of intracellular potassium. The increased nitrogen excretion is due to the breakdown of tissue. These changes are a normal response to trauma and in most cases the disturbances are slight and do not require any action. Most patients with a fractured mandible are on a normal diet and fluid intake up to the time of injury and are therefore in normal electrolyte balance. Usually such patients can return to an adequate fluid intake by mouth as soon as the fracture is immobilized and such cases present no fluid balance problems. In conscious patients the fluid intake can be left to the desires of the patient, for normally the kidneys have enormous flexibility of function and can excrete excess salt or fluid from the body. This flexibility, as already stated, is temporarily lost following trauma and operation. Intravenous fluids lack the safeguard of the patient's desire for fluid and therefore the amount administered has to be accurately assessed by the surgeon.

In a patient unable to swallow, due to a severe mandibular fracture, considerable dehydration can occur in 24–48 hours, especially in elderly patients. If the patient is capable of taking fluid by mouth, it is unnecessary to employ any other route, but if for some reason the patient cannot swallow, enteral or parenteral fluid therapy must be instituted.

Enteral Fluid Therapy.—Enteral fluid therapy is effected by gravitating fluid into the stomach via a transnasal gastric drip, and 4 volumes of 5 per cent dextrose solution to 1 volume of isotonic saline meets the body needs in dehydration. A Ryle's tube constructed of Portex is less irritating to the gastric mucosa than the rubber variety.

Parenteral Fluid Therapy.—Parenteral fluid therapy is administered by an intravenous drip and the greatest risk with this form of therapy is that of overloading the patient with water while the normal kidney flexibility of function is temporarily impaired as a result of the trauma and/or operation. It is exceptional for patients who have sustained a fractured mandible to require intravenous fluid in the postoperative period in the absence of some complication such as protracted unconsciousness, though intravenous blood or other fluid may have to be given immediately following the accident if the patient is shocked. As already stated, shock is rare following fracture of the mandible and if present is usually due to some associated injury. In all instances patients should revert to oral fluid and feeding as soon as possible.

3. The Late Postoperative Care of Mandibular Fractures

Period of Immobilization.—A mandibular fracture occurring in a normal healthy adult requires about 5 weeks' immobilization after the fragments have been adequately reduced. Fractures in children unite in 3–4 weeks, while in the elderly patient, or when the fracture is infected, a period of 6–7 weeks may be required.

Testing of Union and Removal of Fixation.—When it is considered that the fracture should be united the fixation is dismantled sufficiently to allow the fracture site to be tested by gentle movement across it, and if union is satisfactory the fixation is removed.

When direct wiring has been employed it is usually necessary to remove all the wiring in order to test the fracture, but if eyelet wiring has been used it is sufficient to remove the tie wires. In the case of cap splints the locking plates are unscrewed and connecting bars removed in order to test fracture sites, and pin fixation apparatus can be disconnected for the same purpose.

Gunning splints have to be removed entirely before testing the fracture and, therefore, difficulty arises if the fracture requires further immobilization.

Where bone-plating or transosseous wires have been employed these are, of course, left in situ.

If the fracture is satisfactorily united the fixation apparatus is removed in the case of direct and eyelet wiring, cap splints, Gunning splints, and external pin fixation. Wiring, direct or eyelet, is removed by sectioning the wire with suitable cutters and unwinding it.

Peralveolar and circumferential wires are removed by cutting one end close to the gum and pulling on the opposite end of wire. No anaesthetic is necessary, but it is essential to cut the wire cleanly, for a jagged end of wire causes pain as it is pulled through the tissues. The mouth should be cleaned with antiseptic such as 1 per cent hibitane solution before pulling out the wire to avoid introducing infection deep into the tissues. It is helpful as an additional safeguard against infection to administer an antibiotic such as 1 mega unit of fortified procaine penicillin at this time.

Cap splints are removed with an old pair of upper Reid forceps. One blade is placed on the edge of the splint near the gingival margin and the other blade on the occlusal surface of the splint. The handles of the forceps are approximated to squeeze the two blades together and the underlying copper cement is cracked. This manœuvre is carried out all round the splint and when it is loose it is lifted off the teeth. The residual black copper cement should be removed as soon as possible as it tends to get excessively hard when bathed in saliva for any length of time. Special care should be taken to remove copper cement from the occlusal surfaces of the teeth, for its presence may derange the bite and cause the patient to adopt a bite of convenience. This tends to throw strain on the newly healed fracture. Extra-oral pins are removed by gripping each pin with heavy pliers and removing it with a rotatory, pulling movement. The skin surrounding the pins should be well cleaned with an antiseptic before removing them to avoid infection.

Adjustment of Occlusion.—Little adjustment of the occlusion is required when direct or eyelet wiring has been employed as the cusps are placed in their correct position under direct vision at the time of immobilization of the fracture.

Some slight adjustment to the occlusion is required, however, when cap splints have been employed, for no matter how accurately they have been constructed there is, of necessity, a layer of splint metal and a layer of cement over the cusp of each tooth incorporated in the splint. Slight derangement of the occlusion can often be overcome by allowing the patient to masticate normally, for usually there is sufficient elasticity in the recently healed fracture to allow the occlusion to correct itself.

More gross abnormalities of the occlusion are treated by selective grinding of the cusps. Special problems arise when only a small number of teeth is present in either jaw, for the patient tends to assume a bite of convenience which imposes a strain across the recently healed fracture line causing it to become mobile again. Such cases should be fitted with partial upper and lower dentures as soon as possible to stabilize the bite. Patients with fractures of the edentulous mandible can seldom wear their original lower dentures and new plates are required when the fracture is healed.

Mobilization of the Temporomandibular Joint.—Patients seldom have any difficulty in moving their temporomandibular joints following a protracted period of immobilization of the mandible, and usually no special treatment is required on removing the fixation beyond encouraging movement. However, if an intracapsular fracture is present or if the fracture in the condylar region could constitute a hazard to the restoration of full mobility of the joint, the fixation should be designed to allow movement of the temporomandibular joints, while fractures elsewhere in the mandible are adequately immobilized. The most common injury where such measures are desirable is the midline or lateral-to-midline fracture associated with fractures in both condylar regions. In such cases the fracture of the body can be immobilized by cap splints, bone plating, or transosseous wiring while the joints are allowed to function normally. Following severe fractures in the condylar region the patient may have some clicking and grating of the joint, but it is surprising how seldom such patients complain of symptoms related to the joint.

Anaesthesia and Parasthesia of the Lower Lip.—If the mandibular nerve is involved in the fracture the damage may take the form of a neurapraxia or neurotmesis and the period for recovery of sensation will, of course, depend on the nature and degree of the damage to the nerve. A neurapraxia usually recovers in about 6 weeks, but a neurotmesis may take 18 months. Following severe damage to the nerve complete recovery may not occur and the patient will complain of a slightly altered sensation on the affected side. However, some degree of sensation in the lip always occurs as the area of the lower lip supplied by the mandibular nerve has an accessory nerve-supply from C2 and 3. The lingual nerve is seldom damaged in civilian-type mandibular fractures but if the nerve is severed sensation in the anterior two-thirds of the tongue is seldom re-established.

Viability of Damaged Teeth.—Teeth subjected to trauma at the time of accident should be kept under observation and their vitality tested for death of the pulp may occur as a late complication.

Gingivitis.—The condition of the gingivae is surprisingly good following the removal of well made cap splints, and provided that oral hygiene is maintained during immobilization with direct or eyelet wiring the condition of the gums remains good. Occasionally, however, the gum may grow over the wires and this makes it more uncomfortable for the patient when they are being removed.

CHAPTER IX

FRACTURES OF THE MANDIBLE IN CHILDREN

FRACTURES of the mandible are uncommon in children owing to the fact that the bone is resilient at this age and considerable force is required to effect a fracture. For the same reason, it is only in young children with relatively soft springy bone that the greenstick-type fracture occurs and this is most common at the neck of the condyle.

The general principles of reduction and fixation of mandibular fractures in children are essentially similar to those in adults, but there are some additional factors which must be taken into consideration when treating these cases.

1. There may be interference with mandibular growth as a result of the injury or the subsequent treatment. The most important growth centre which may be affected in this way is the condylar growth centre and the question of the treatment of fractures in this region occurring before mandibular growth is complete has already been discussed in the section on condylar fractures.

Interference with the normal growth of the mandible is also caused if unerupted permanent teeth are lost, for the alveolus does not grow normally in the areas affected. This damage may occur as a result of the original injury or erupted teeth may have to be removed as a prophylactic measure to prevent infection.

2. Unerupted and partially erupted teeth of the permanent dentition or the presence of loose deciduous teeth may complicate the techniques selected for the immobilization of the fragments.

If teeth are to be used for immobilization the technique for fixation must vary according to the number and mobility of teeth available for this purpose.

a. If the deciduous teeth are unerupted, or an inadequate number are available, or if they have been loosened as a result of the accident and have to be extracted, an overall Gunning-type splint is very effective. Only a lower Gunning-type splint in the form of a trough is required and this is lined with black gutta percha and retained by two circumferential wires.

b. If a complete deciduous dentition of firm teeth is available, either cap splints or interdental eyelet wiring can be used.

c. If many deciduous teeth have been shed or are extremely mobile and the permanent teeth are not erupted, an overall Gunning-type splint should be used as in (*a*), after all loose teeth have been extracted.

d. If a few firm deciduous teeth and some permanent teeth are present, cap splints can be used.

e. If all the deciduous teeth are lost and one or more permanent teeth are adequately erupted and present on each fragment, cap splints may be used.

f. If an adequate number of fully erupted permanent teeth are present, arch bar or eyelet wiring is possible.

If cap splints are used it is helpful to reinforce the cement with which they are attached to the teeth with a circumferential wire tied over the splint. This is especially useful if the teeth incorporated in the splint are not fully erupted.

3. Owing to the presence of unerupted teeth, transosseous wiring should be used with caution for fear of damaging developing teeth. For the same reason extra-oral pin fixation and bone plating are contra-indicated.

4. Some imperfection in reduction can be accepted, for slight derangements of the occlusion will be corrected when the teeth erupt.

5. Mandibular fractures in children heal more rapidly than adults and fractures are often firmly united in 3 weeks. If at the time the fracture is first seen the fragments are firm, but not perfectly reduced, it is as well to accept some slight imperfection in the reduction rather than refracture the mandible and possibly damage developing teeth. Normal growth and eruption of teeth will usually compensate quite satisfactorily for any slight lack of alinement of the fragments.

6. The presence of unerupted teeth sometimes makes the radiological diagnosis of a crack fracture difficult.

7. Children are usually good patients, but it is helpful to carry out the necessary reduction and fixation under general anaesthesia.

CHAPTER X

COMPLICATIONS

COMPLICATIONS arising as a result of a fracture of the mandible are extremely rare providing the fracture has been competently treated. Possible complications are:—

1. Anaesthesia of the lower lip as a result of neurapraxia or neurotmesis of the mandibular nerve. This is the most common complication of fracture of the body of the mandible and the recovery rate depends upon the nature of the original damage to the nerve. A neurapraxia will usually recover completely in about a month to six weeks, but if the nerve is severed recovery is protracted to about a year or eighteen months and may, in some instances, never recover fully. As already stated, some recovery of sensation in the lower lip always occurs owing to the fact that the area supplied by the mandibular nerve has an accessory nerve-supply from C2 and C3. If anaesthesia is present the patient should be reassured and the condition kept under observation. The patient should be warned of the danger of burning the lower lip with hot drinks or cigarettes.

2. Scars.—Many mandibular fractures have an associated soft-tissue injury and provided these wounds are carefully cleaned and sutured minimal scarring occurs. At first all scars tend to be red and feel lumpy, but with time they improve and become less obvious. Massage of the scar by the patient using lanoline is helpful in this respect. Occasionally keloid or hypertrophic scarring occurs and produces an ugly deformity. Such scars tend to improve with time, but occasionally a plastic surgical rearrangement of the scar may help to improve it and occasionally treatment with low dosage X-rays will improve its appearance. Wounds contaminated with road dirt, especially tar, produce ugly pigmented scars which can only be improved by surgical excision of the scar. To avoid this late complication, wounds should be cleaned of all debris before suturing. A toothbrush dipped in 1 per cent Cetavlon is a useful instrument for this purpose.

3. Derangement of the Occlusion.—Provided the treatment of the fracture is competent only a minor degree of occlusal derangement occurs. If minimal derangement of the occlusion is present when the fixation is first removed the patient should be allowed to use the jaw and this usually results in the bite correcting itself. Persistence of a traumatogenic occlusion is treated by selective grinding of the cusps.

Gross occlusal derangement in a neglected fracture may require re-fracture of the mandible and correction of the abnormality, or, if this is not considered desirable, selective extraction of teeth may be necessary.

If the patient is edentulous it is usually necessary to reline or remake the dentures at the completion of treatment.

4. Non-union (*see* p. 66).—Provided the fracture has been treated competently, non-union is practically unknown. However, if a tooth has been left in the fracture line, or the fracture is infected from some other cause, or if immobilization has been inadequate, non-union or greatly delayed union may result. Fibrous union may also occur if a patient with a minimal number of teeth adopts a bite of convenience shortly after the fixation is removed and produces great stress across the recently healed fracture line. To avoid this complication such patients should have their occlusion corrected by the provision of partial dentures immediately after the fixation is removed. Some cases of delayed or non-union can be cured by removing any impediment to normal healing such as a tooth in the fracture line and then freshening the opposing bone-ends surgically and immobilizing the fragments again. If the non-union has been present many months and the bone-ends are eburnated a bone-graft may be necessary.

5. **Derangements of the Temporomandibular Joint.**—Mobilization of the temporomandibular joints occurs surprisingly easily following the removal of mandibular–maxillary fixation, even if immobilization has been considerably protracted. This is true even when severe damage has occurred in the condylar neck region. However, when treating such fractures it is prudent to release the mandibular–maxillary fixation at some stage of the immobilization period to ascertain whether the temporo-mandibular joints are functioning satisfactorily. If they are moving normally the mandibular–maxillary fixation is reassembled. To facilitate such periodic examinations of the continuing function of the joints the fixation in such cases should be designed to facilitate release of the mandibular–maxillary fixation, i.e., eyelet wiring, etc., should be avoided if possible and cap splints substituted. If a tendency to limitation of movement is noted steps must be taken to mobilize the joints even if this necessitates a change of fixation. If such a complication is anticipated, as for instance in the case of an intracapsular fracture, the fixation technique should be designed to enable the joints to remain mobilized throughout treatment. This can be effected by using an overall cap splint in the mandible or by bone plating of the fracture if the patient is edentulous.

Even following severe fracture dislocation of the condyles a good functional result can be anticipated and, although clicking and grating of the joints may sometimes occur, it is rare for a patient to complain of symptoms in the area.

6. **Deformity of the Mandible and Malposition of the Fragments.**— Provided the reduction and other treatment have been adequately per-formed no obvious deformity of the mandible should result.

Remodelling of the bone occurs comparatively rapidly and even follow-ing a severe comminuted fracture it is surprising how soon the radio-graphs will reveal a relatively normal mandibular contour. A fracture at the angle with upward and forward displacement of the posterior fragment also eventually becomes corrected. This raises an interesting point as to whether it is justifiable to perform a lengthy and more complicated operation on an ill patient, such as a lower-border transosseous wiring of multiple fragments, in order to achieve perfect reduction if a more simple and rapid technique giving a less satisfactory position will achieve a similar result by remodelling in a matter of months.

One situation where remodelling of the bone does not restore the normal mandibular contour is in a fracture occurring to one side of the genial tubercles. Failure to reposition the fragments accurately results in the backwardly displaced fragment remaining in this position even though adequate bony union has occurred, and this gives the patient a marked asymmetrical appearance.

7. **Infection.**—Infection of the bone resulting in necrosis or osteomyelitis of the mandible is most rare. Infection is obviously possible if, for instance, a tooth or root has been left in the fracture line and it is sometimes seen in pathological fractures occurring as a result of some benign or malignant neoplasm. Extreme lowering of the patient's local or general resistance may also predispose to infection as a complication of fracture, but in the normal straightforward civilian-type fracture which has been competently managed infection is most rare. To avoid possible infection it is prudent to carry out mandibular–maxillary fixation in all fractures which are compound into the mouth, for movement of the mandible tends to pump infection down the fracture line. There are very few fractures involving the body of the mandible which can safely be left without any fixation. It is also important to administer a short course of antibiotics such as 1 mega unit of fortified procaine penicillin daily for 4 days at the start of treatment to prevent the fracture haematoma becoming infected.

Some of the most severe infections of fracture sites are seen as a result of injudicious surgical interference, such as a lower border wiring of a fracture already infected, and no foreign material such as wire or bone plates should be introduced if there is any suspicion that the site of fracture is already infected.

8. **Actinomycosis.**—A rare complication of fractures of the mandible is actinomycosis. The infection occurs as a late complication and usually presents as a moderate swelling beneath the mandible which is not particularly painful or inflamed. Diagnosis is made by aspiration and bacteriological examination of the pus, and treatment is by protracted (about 6 weeks) use of antibiotics such as 1 mega unit of penicillin daily. The condition is most commonly seen following fractures in the incisor area with possible introduction of calculus into the fracture site. Actinomycosis should be suspected in the case of any low grade inflammatory swelling occurring as a late complication of a mandibular fracture.

9. **Gingivitis.**—Gingivitis, as a late complication following the use of splints or eyelet or arch wiring, is most unusual in the absence of a pre-existing paradontal condition.

10.—**Traumatic Myositis Ossificans of the Masseter.**—Traumatic myositis ossificans is occasionally found in the masseter muscle after either repeated minor or a solitary instance of major trauma over the masseter. It is believed that haematoma formation occurs in the masseter muscle and that eventually the haematoma becomes ossified. The usual story is of trauma over the masseter muscle followed by increasing trismus over a period of about 6 weeks, and eventually the trismus becomes complete. Attempts by both patient and clinician to open the jaw are fruitless and a bony bar may sometimes be palpated intra-orally in the masseter region. In a case seen by the author this bar extended to the zygomatic bone. Difficulty is experienced in demonstrating the bony mass radiographically, but the nature of the lesion is readily seen on tomograms.

Treatment is by excision of the bony mass, but sometimes the condition may recur. Few cases have been reported in the literature and this is surprising in view of the fact that owing to its exposed position the masseter must often be subjected to trauma. It would seem that some additional factor or factors must be involved in the development of myositis ossificans, but at present the exact aetiology of the condition is unknown.

CHAPTER XI

MAL-UNION: DELAYED UNION AND NON-UNION

Mal-union.—Post-reduction radiographs must always be taken and should these reveal an unacceptable malposition of the fragments this should be corrected as soon as possible.

Cases where inadequate reduction has resulted in gross deformity of the face or derangement of the occlusion are sometimes referred when the fragments are already united. These may be treated by surgical refracture and immobilization, or if this is not considered desirable selective extractions can be carried out to improve the occlusion. Facial deformity may be improved with the aid of buccal inlays, autograft or allelograft onlays, osteotomy or ostectomy.

As already stated, the mandible has an impressive capacity for re-modelling itself and attempting to return to its normal configuration. Slight imperfections in the alinement of the fragments may therefore be accepted in the knowledge that in time correction will occur by the bone remodelling. This is especially true of the comminuted type of fracture and in such cases it is unnecessary to position each fragment accurately into its original position, for in time the various fragments will consolidate and the mandible remodel to a relatively normal contour.

Delayed and Non-union.—

Delayed Union.—If the time taken for a mandibular fracture to unite is unduly protracted it is referred to as a case of 'delayed union'. This is an arbitrary and artificial term, for fractures unite at different rates. For instance, fractures in children unite rapidly, while in elderly patients delayed union is to be expected.

Delayed healing of fractures in elderly patients may be caused not only by senile osteoporosis secondary to endocrine changes associated with a calcium deficiency, but also by a deficiency of vitamin C.

Non-union.—Non-union means that the fracture is not only not united but will not unite on its own. Radiographs show rounding off and sclerosis of the bone-ends, a condition referred to as 'eburnation'.

Under the term 'non-union' is also included the condition of fibrous union, where the fracture has not consolidated but where the bone-ends are joined by fibrous tissue which gives a moderate degree of stability.

Non-union or greatly delayed union may occur when the fracture becomes infected, when there is inadequate immobilization, where apposition of the bone-ends is unsatisfactory, and where the blood-supply to the bone-ends is inadequate. It is a condition easier to prevent than cure and if fractures of the mandible are adequately treated non-union does not occur. Antibiotics in the early stages of treatment will prevent infection of the fracture haematoma as will the removal of devitalized teeth from the fracture line. Satisfactory reduction with adequate immobilization of the fragments for the requisite period of time will then give a uniformly good result. As already stated the movement of a mobile mandible tends to pump infection into any fracture compounded into the mouth and where such conditions obtain it is prudent to immobilize the mandible in order to prevent infection.

The mandible has a great tendency to unite following fracture provided it is not actively hindered from doing so and in parts of the world where treatment is not available it is salutary to observe how many completely untreated mandibular fractures eventually cure themselves. Some of the worst cases of non-union seen have been brought about by ill-judged surgical interference in the form of lower border transosseous wiring of an already infected fracture site. The resulting necrosis may produce a disastrous result.

The adoption by the patient of a bite of convenience which throws a strain across an apparently healed fracture may eventually result in a fibrous union. It is therefore important to provide such a patient with a satisfactory occlusion by fitting suitable dentures as soon as possible.

Some pathological fractures fail to unite as for example in active malignant disease of the mandible, osteoradionecrosis, and Albers-Schoenberg or marble bone disease.

Excessive bone loss following a gunshot injury will also result in a non-union.

Treatment.—A moderate delay in union is treated by prolonging the period of immobilization. However, if union of a fracture is excessively protracted the fracture line should be explored surgically and any obvious impediment to healing such as a devitalized tooth or sequestrum removed. The bone-ends are then freshened and the wound closed, following which the jaw is immobilized again. If this is not successful within an adequate period of time a bone-graft is necessary.

If radiographs of a non-union show marked eburnation of the bone-ends or there is excessive bone loss, a bone-graft will be required. It is, of course, important that before contemplating a bone-graft the site should be completely free of infection or the graft will be rejected.

Occasionally an elderly infirm patient is seen with a fibrous non-union which is apparently causing no great inconvenience and in such a case it is prudent to accept the position. However, the majority of cases of non-union of the mandible require active treatment.

CHAPTER XII

FRACTURES WITH GROSS COMMINUTION OF BONE AND LOSS OF HARD AND SOFT TISSUE

TREATMENT of the so-called 'gunshot'-type fracture of the mandible presents a difficult problem in view of the loss of both hard and soft tissue. The reason for this extensive tissue destruction is that the missile shatters the teeth and bone on impact, and imparts to these particles a velocity which propels them through the tissues, so producing an extensive 'explosive' exit wound, though the entry wound of the missile may be comparatively small. Extensive comminution of the mandible results and both hard and soft tissue is lost.

Such extensive injuries of the mandible require protracted treatment and the management of such cases can be divided into six main phases.

1. Immediate Post-traumatic Phase.—The patient is not particularly shocked as a result of such an injury but haemorrhage may be severe and there is an immediate risk of respiratory obstruction from the tongue falling back owing to the loss of its anterior skeletal attachment. Immediate steps must be taken to control the tongue with a suture and care must be taken when transporting such cases to see that they are not laid on their back as they will rapidly suffocate. Stretcher cases should be laid face downwards with their face over the end of the stretcher and their forehead supported on a bandage tied between the two handles of the stretcher, or they can be carried lying on their side. Either position ensures that the tongue falls forwards and blood and saliva drain out of the mouth.

Ambulatory cases are made to hold their face downwards and forwards. These patients are not usually in much pain and powerful analgesics such as morphine should not be administered as they depress the cough reflex and respiratory centre. A 'doped' patient may inadvertently suffocate during this critical period. There is also the risk of morphia not being immediately absorbed if the patient is shocked and several doses of this analgesic may be administered with little effect and are suddenly released into the blood-stream some hours later when resuscitatory measures are instituted, resulting in morphine poisoning.

2. Preliminary Surgery.—When surgical facilities are available a tracheostomy is performed to control the airway and a débridement of the wound is carried out. The remaining soft and hard tissue is returned to its correct position and if sufficient mandibular bone remains mandibular-maxillary fixation is effected by any of the techniques already discussed in treating civilian-type fractures. No attempt is made at this stage to close gaps in hard or soft tissue resulting from actual loss of tissue. However, to prevent the exposed bone-ends becoming infected skin is sutured to mucous membrane and plans are made to repair the soft and hard tissue at a later date.

3. Saliva Shield Phase.—While the patient is waiting to have the soft tissue repair effected the gaping facial wound causes extreme distress. Saliva dribbles down the chest and the patient is unable to drink, speak, smoke, etc. In order to make life more tolerable a saliva shield is constructed. This consists of an acrylic cover lined with black gutta percha which fits over the space caused by the missing tissue and is held in place with an attachment tied round the back of the patient's head and neck. This device enables the patient to eat and speak and it is worn until the gap in the facial soft tissues is closed by surgery.

4. Soft Tissue Repair.—Surgical repair of the soft tissue defect is effected with pedicle grafts or rotation flaps.

5. Bone-grafting.—After the soft tissues have been repaired the bone lost is restored with bone-grafts from the ribs or iliac crest.

6. Restoration of Normal Mandibular Contour.—Even when both hard and soft tissue have been replaced the patient frequently requires further surgery to improve the appearance. The usual residual deformity is a loss of chin prominence and this can be corrected by a buccal inlay and prosthesis or an onlay or even a bilateral osteotomy and bilateral bone-grafts.

Throughout treatment the techniques used to immobilize the bone fragments are similar to those already described for the treatment of so-called 'civilian-type' mandibular fractures.

BIBLIOGRAPHY

ADAMS, W. M., and ADAMS, L. H. (1956), 'Internal Wire Fixation of Fractures. 15-year Follow-up', *Amer. J. Surg.*, **92**, 12.

ALTY, H. M. (1963), 'Atrophy of the Mandible and Spontaneous Fracture', *Brit. dent. J.*, **114**, 188.

ANDREWS, J. (1968), 'Maxillo-facial Trauma in Vietnam', *J. oral Surg.*, **26**, 457.

ARENTZ, R. (1967), 'Severe Facial Fractures in a Haemophiliac', *Ibid.*, **25**, 358.

ATTERBURY, R. A., and PANAGOPOULOS, A. P. (1959), 'Management of Multiple, Compound, Comminuted Mandibular Fracture in a 3 Year Old Child', *Oral Surg.*, **12**, 421.

BATTERSBY, T. G. (1966), 'Plating of Mandibular Fractures', *Brit. J. oral Surg.*, **4**, 194.

— — (1967), 'Sequel to Gunshot Wound of Face', *Ibid.*, **5**, 117.

BATTLE, R. J. V. (1953), 'War History of Plastic Surgery in the Army', *History of the Second World War* (*Surgery*), p. 341. London: H.M.S.O.

BECKER, W. H. (1950), 'Transosseous Wiring Fixation of Condylar Fractures with Intrafacial Incision', *Oral Surg.*, **3**, 284.

— — (1952), 'Open Reduction of Mandibular Fractures', *Ibid.*, **5**, 447.

BISI, R. H. (1973), 'The Management of Mandibular Fractures in Edentulous Patients by Intramedullary Pinning', *Laryngoscope, St Louis*, **83**, 22.

BLEVINS, C., and GORES, R. J. (1961), 'Fractures of the Mandibular Condyloid Process: Results of Conservative Treatment in 140 Patients', *J. oral Surg.*, **19**, 392.

BLOCK, C., and others (1972), 'Use of a Metal Intra-osseous Fixation Device for Treatment of Fractures of Atrophic Edentulous Mandibles', *J. Sth. Calif. dent. Ass.*, **40**, 996.

BOOTH, N. A. (1953), 'Complications associated with Treatment of Traumatic Injuries of the Oral Cavity: Aspiration of Teeth', *Ibid.*, **11**, 242.

BOSCO, H. F. (1960), 'Reconstruction of Mandible following Bone Loss due to Osteomyelitis in the Line of Fracture', *Oral Surg.*, **13**, 663.

BRADNUM, P. (1960), 'Improved Method of Fixation of Silver Splints', *Brit. dent. J.*, **108**, 302.

BRAMLEY, P., and FORBES, A. (1960), 'A Case of Progressive Hemiatrophy presenting with Spontaneous Fractures of the Lower Jaw', *Brit. med. J.*, **1**, 1476.

BROADBENT, T. R. (1954), 'Mandibular Condyle Fractures', *Plastic reconstr. Surg.*, **14**, 148.

BROMIDGE, M. R. (1971), 'Severe Compound Comminuted Fractures of the Mandible', *Brit. J. oral Surg.*, **9**, 29.

BRONS, R. (1970), *Stabiele Interne Fixatie bij Corpus Mandibulae-Frakturen*. Groningen: Niemeyer.

BROWN, J. B., FRYER, M. P., and McDOWEL, F. (1949), 'Internal Wire-pin Immobilization of Jaw Fractures', *Plastic Reconstr. Surg.*, **4**, 30.

BROWN, J. B. and McDOWELL, F. (1942), 'Internal Wire Fixation for Fractures of the Jaw: Preliminary Report', *Surg. Gynec. Obstet.*, **74**, 227.

BURCH, R. J., and others (1958), 'Method of Reduction for Impacted and Partially Malunited Fractures of the Jaws', *J. oral Surg.*, **16**, 336.

BUXTON, J. L. D., PARFITT, G. J., and MACGREGOR, A. N. (1941), 'Arch Wires for the Immobilization of Fractures of the Mandible', *Brit. dent. J.*, **71**, 295.

BYRNE, R. P. (1972), 'Occult Fracture of the Odontoid Process: Report of Case', *J. oral Surg.*, **30**, 684.

CALHOUN, N. R., and PERKINS, R. L. (1958), 'Compound, Comminuted Fracture of Body of Mandible', *J. oral Surg.*, **16**, 510.

CHARLTON, H. (1967), 'An Occipital Air Support for use with the Ellis "Halo" ', *Brit. J. oral Surg.*, **5**, 167.

CLARKSON, P. W., WILSON, T. H. H., and LAWRIE, R. S. (1946), 'Treatment of 1,000 Jaw Fractures', *Brit. dent. J.*, **80**, 69.

COHEN, B. (1968), 'Management of Comminuted Mandibular Fractures', *J. oral Surg.*, **26**, 537.

CURRAN, J. B., and others (1972), 'Diplopia as a Sign of Basal Skull Fracture accompanying a Fractured Mandible: Report of Case', *J. oral Surg.*, **30**, 845.

DE'CHAMPLAIN, R. W. (1973) 'Mandibular Reconstruction', *J. oral Surg.*, **31**, 448.

DES PREZ, J. D., and KIEHN, C. L. (1959), 'Methods of Reconstruction following Resection of Anterior Oral Cavity and Mandible for Malignancy', *Plast. reconstr. Surg.*, **24**, 238.

DINGMAN, R. O., and ALLING, C. C. (1954), 'Open Reduction and Internal Wire Fixation of Maxillo-facial Fractures', *J. oral Surg.*, **12**, 140.

—— and HARDING, R. L. (1951), 'Treatment of Mal-union of Fractures of the Facial Bones', *Plastic reconstr. Surg.*, **7**, 505.

—— and NATVIG, P. (1964), *Surgery of Facial Fractures*. London: Sanders.

DITCHFIELD, A. (1960), 'Interosseous Wiring of Mandibular Fractures: A Follow-up of 50 Cases', *Brit. J. plast. Surg.*, **13**, 146.

DONOFF, R. B., and others (1973), 'Management of Condylar Fractures in Patients with Cervical Spine Injury: Report of Cases', *J. oral Surg.*, **31**, 130.

ELLIS, D., and others (1972), 'Fracture of the Mandible in a 5-year-old Infant', *Oral Surg.*, **33**, 348.

FARISH, S. E. (1972), 'Iatrogenic Fracture of the Coronoid Process: Report of Case', *J. oral Surg.*, **30**, 848.

FICKLING, B. W. (1946), 'Advances in Construction and Use of Splints in Treatment', *Brit. dent. J.*, **80**, 8.

FORDYCE, G. L. (1957), 'Pyriform Aperture Wiring in the Treatment of Mandibular Fractures', *Brit. J. plast. Surg.*, **9**, 304.

FREIHOFER, H. P. M. (1973), 'Experiences with Intra-oral Transosseous Wiring of Mandibular Fractures', *J. max. fac. Surg.*, **1**, 248.

FRY, W. K. (1929), 'Fractures of the Mandible in and Posterior to the Molar Region', *Proc. R. Soc. Med.*, **22**, 37.

—— SHEPHERD, P. P., McLEOD, A. C., and PARFITT, G. J. (1943), *The Dental Treatment of Maxillo-facial Injuries*. Oxford: Blackwell.

FRYER, M. P. (1971), 'Evaluation of Internal Wire Pin Fixation of Mandibular Fractures', *Surgery Gynec. Obstet.*, **132**, 19.

GARIULO, E. A. (1973), 'Use of Titanium Mesh and Autogenous Bone Marrow in the Repair of a Non-united Mandibular Fracture: Report of Case and Review of the Literature', *J. oral Surg.*, **31**, 371.

GEORGIADE, N. G., ed. (1969), *Plastic and Maxillo-facial Trauma Symposium*. St. Louis: Mosby.

GILHUUS-MOE, O. (1971), 'Fractures of the Mandibular Condyle in the Growth Period', *Acta odont. scand.*, **29**, 53.

GILLIES, H. D. (1920), *Plastic Surgery of the Face*. London: Oxford University Press.

GOODSELL, O. (1964), 'Traumatic Myositis Ossificans of the Masseter Muscle', *Brit. J. oral Surg.*, **2**, 137.

GORACY, E. S., and others (1971), 'Traumatic Refracture of the Mandible', *Oral Surg.*, **32**, 378.

GORDON, S. (1957), 'A Prosthetic Mandibular Head: Case Report', *Plastic reconstr. Surg.*, **20**, 62.

GORMAN, J. M., and others (1972), 'An Impacted Mandibular Fracture', *Brit. J. oral Surg.*, **10**, 95.

GRATTAN, E. (1972), 'Patterns, Causes and Prevention of Facial Injury in Car Occupants', *Proc. R. Soc. Med.*, **65**, 913.

GUNNING, T. B. (1866), 'The Treatment of Fractures of the Lower Jaw by Interdental Splints', *N.Y. med. J.*, **3**, 433.

HALAZONETIS, J. A. (1968), 'The Weak Regions of the Mandible', *Brit. J. oral Surg.*, **6**, 37.

HANRATTY, W. J., and NAEVE, H. F. (1964), 'Actinomycosis with Pathologic Fracture of Mandible', *Oral Surg.*, **18**, 303.

HARNISCH, H. (1959), 'Five-year Statistics of Jaw Fractures', *Zahnärztl. Prax.*, **10**, 126.

HENDRIX, J. H., and others (1959), 'Open Reduction of Mandibular Condyle; A Clinical and Experimental Study', *Plastic reconstr. Surg.*, **23**, 283.

HOLDEN, M. (1968), 'An Unusual Complication arising during the Treatment of a Mandibular Fracture', *Brit. J. oral Surg.*, **6**, 93.

HOOPES, J. E., and others (1970), 'Operative Treatment of Fractures of the Mandibular Condyle in Children using the Post-auricular Approach', *Plastic reconstr. Surg.*, **46**, 357.

HOWE, G. L., and WILSON, J. S. P. (1964), 'Traumatic Arterio-venous Aneurysm occurring as a Complication of a Mandibular Fracture: Case Report', *Ibid.*, **2**, 54.

HUELKE, D. F., and BURDI, A. R. (1964), 'Location of Mandibular Fractures related to Teeth and Edentulous Regions', *J. oral Surg.*, **22**, 396.

— — and others (1962), 'Association between Mandibular Fractures and Site of Trauma, Dentition and Age', *Ibid.*, **20**, 478.

HUESTON, J. T. (1959), 'Surgical Exposure of the Dislocated Mandibular Condyle', *Brit. J. plast. Surg.*, **12**, 275.

HUNGERFORD, R. W., and MUNSAT, T. L. (1965), 'Mandibular Fracture and Myotonic Dystrophy', *Oral Surg.*, **18**, 121.

HUNSUCK, E. (1967), 'A Method of Intraoral Open Reduction of Fractured Mandibles', *J. oral Surg.*, **25**, 233.

HUNTER, K. M. (1972), 'Midline and Condylar Fracture in an 18-month-old Child', *Aust. dent. J.*, **17**, 373.

HUT, M. (1960), 'Methods and Appliances for the Reduction and Fixation of Fractures of the Facial Bones', *Int. dent. J., Lond.*, **10**, 468.

IRBY, W. B. (1958), 'Correction of Malreduced Fractures of Mandible at Angles', *Oral Surg.*, **11**, 26.

—— (1969), 'Facial Injuries in Military Combat. Intermediate Care', *J. oral Surg.*, **27**, 548.

JACOBSEN, P. U. (1972), 'Unilateral Overgrowth and Remodelling Processes after Fracture of the Mandibular Condyle: A Longitudinal Radiographic Study', *Scand. J. dent. Res.*, **80**, 68.

JAMES, W. W., and FICKLING, B. W. (1940), *Injuries of Face and Jaws.* London: Bale & Staples.

JOHNSON, G. B. (1962), 'Multiple Severe Automotive Injuries. Evaluation and Management', *N. C. med. J.*, **22**, 335.

JONES, R. WATSON (1952), *Fractures and Joint Injuries*, 4th ed., vol. 1. Edinburgh: Livingstone.

KAZANJIAN, V. H., and CONVERSE, J. M. (1949), *The Surgical Treatment of Facial Fractures.* Baltimore: Williams & Wilkins.

———— (1959), *The Surgical Treatment of Facial Injuries*, 2nd ed. Baltimore: Williams & Wilkins.

KEEN, R. R. (1971), 'Mandibular Fracture in a Small Child', *Ill. dent. J.*, **40**, 87.

KENIRY, A. J. (1971), 'A Survey of Jaw Fracture in Children', *Brit. J. oral Surg.*, **8**, 213.

KHOSLA, M., and others (1971), 'Mandibular Fractures in Children and their Management', *J. oral Surg.*, **29**, 116.

KIEHN, C. L., and others (1961), 'Management of Fractures of the Mandibular Condyle', *J. Trauma*, **1**, 279.

KILLEY, H. C. (1968), 'Maxillo-facial Injuries', *Hospital Med.*, **2**, 917.

KLINE, S. N. (1973), 'Lateral Compression in the Treatment of Mandibular Fractures', *J. oral Surg.*, **31**, 182.

KROMER, H. (1952), Reprinted from *Norske Tandlaegeforen. Tid.*

—— (1953), 'Teeth in the Line of Fracture: A Conception of the Problem based on a Review of 690 Jaw Fractures', *Brit. dent. J.*, **95**, 43.

KWAPIS, B. W., and others (1973), 'Surgical Correction of a Mal-united Condylar Fracture in a Child', *J. oral Surg.*, **31**, 465.

LAL, D., and others (1959), 'Management of Fractures of Lower Jaw in Children', *Oral Surg.*, **12**, 1413.

LAPIDOT, A. (1962), 'Clinical Survey of Fractures of the Mandible with Special Reference to Early and Controlled Mobilization and its Effect on Fracture Union', *Ibid.*, **15**, 518.

LAWS, M. (1967), 'Two Unusual Complications of Fractured Condyles', *Brit. J. oral Surg.*, **5**, 51.

LEAKE, D. (1971), 'Long-term Follow-up of Fractures of the Mandibular Condyle in Children', *Plastic reconstr. Surg.*, **47**, 127.

LE QUESNE, L. P. (1957), *Fluid Balance in Surgical Practice*, 2nd ed. London: Lloyd-Luke.

LEVIN, H. L. (1965), 'Multiple Fractures of the Mandible with Pathological Connotations', *Oral Surg.*, **19**, 179.

LEWIS, G. K., and PERUTSEA, S. C. (1959), 'The Complex Mandibular Fracture', *Amer. J. Surg.*, **97**, 283.

LIGHTERMAN, I., and others (1963), 'Mandibular Fractures Treated with Plastic Polymers', *Arch. Surg., Chicago*, **87**, 868.

LINDSTROM, D. (1960), 'A Comparative Survey of Jaw Fractures during the Years 1948–1958', *Suom. Hammaslääk. Seur. Toim.*, **56**, 16.

LUND, K. (1972), 'Unusual Fracture Dislocation of the Mandibular Condyle in a 6-year-old Child', *Int. J. oral Surg.*, **1**, 53.

LUNDIN, K., and others (1973), 'One Thousand Maxillo-facial and related Fractures of the E.N.T. Clinic in Gothenburg: a 2-year Prospective Study', *Acta otolaryngol.*, **75**, 359.

LUNDQUIST, C. (1960), 'Emergency Treatment of Maxillo-facial Injuries', *Int. dent. J., Lond.*, **10**, 476.

McDOWELL, R., and BROWN, J. B. (1952), 'Internal Fixation of Jaw Fractures', *Arch. Surg., Chicago*, **64**, 665.

MACGREGOR, A. J. (1963), 'Adjustable Locking Plate for Sectional Metal Cap Splints', *Dent. Practit.*, **13**, 341.

— — and FORDYCE, G. (1957), 'The Treatment of Fracture of the Neck of the Mandibular Condyle', *Brit. dent. J.*, **102**, 351.

MACLENNAN, W. D. (1952), 'Consideration of 180 Cases of Typical Fracture of the Mandibular Condylar Process', *Brit. J. plast. Surg.*, **5**, 122.

— — (1956), 'Fractures of the Mandible in Children under the Age of 6 Years', *Ibid.*, **9**, 125.

— — and SIMPSON, W. (1965), 'Treatment of Fractured Mandibular Condylar Process in Children', *Ibid.*, **18**, 423.

MACLEOD, A. C. R., and SHEPHERD, P. R. (1941), 'Cap Splints', *Brit. dent. J.*, **71**, 267.

MALLETT, S. P. (1950), 'Fractures of the Jaw. A Survey of 2124 Cases', *J. Amer. dent. Ass.*, **41**, 657.

MARLETTE, R. H. (1963), 'Submucoperiosteal Wire Fixation of Mandibular Fractures', *J. oral Surg.*, **21**, 409.

MARSDEN, J. L. (1964), 'Fracture of the Mandible due to Radicular and Residual Odontogenic Cysts', *Brit. J. oral Surg.*, **2**, 71.

MAY, M., and others (1972), 'Closed Management of Mandibular Fractures', *Arch. otolaryngol.*, **95**, 53.

— — and others (1973), 'Mandibular Fractures from Civilian Gunshot Wounds: A Study of 20 Cases', *Laryngoscope, St Louis*, **83**, 969.

MERKX, C. A. (1971), 'Treatment of Pseudo Arthrosis of the Mandibular Body by a Sliding Bone Graft', *Arch. Chir. Neerl.*, **23**, 273.

MOONEY, J. W., and others (1972), 'Use of Wire Sutures for Fracture Fixation', *Oral Surg.*, **34**, 21.

MORGAN, E. J. R. (1960), 'Unusual Complication of Fracture of the Neck of the Mandibular Condyle', *Brit. dent. J.*, **108**, 329.

MOWLEM, R., BUXTON, J. L. D., MACGREGOR, A. N., and BARRON, J. N. (1941), 'External Pin Fixation of Fractures of the Mandible', *Lancet*, **2**, 291.

MUŠKA, K. (1968), 'Suspended Fixation of the Mandible', *J. oral Surg.*, **26**, 172.

OBWEGESER, H. L. (1973), 'Another Way of Treating Fractures of the Atrophic Edentulous Mandible', *J. max. fac. Surg.*, **1**, 213.

OIKARINEN, V., and MALMSTROM, M. (1969), 'Jaw Fractures (1284 Cases)', *Suom. Hammaslääk. Seur. Toim.*, **65**, 95.

PANAGOPOULOS, A. P. (1957), 'Management of Fractures of the Jaws in Children', *J. int. Coll. Surg.*, **28**, 806.

— — and MANSUETO, M. D. (1960), 'Treatment of Fractures of the Mandibular Condyloid Process in Children', *Amer. J. Surg.*, **100**, 835.

PAUL, J. K. (1968a), 'Continuous Arch Bar', *J. oral Surg.*, **26**, 114.

— — (1968b), 'Intraoral Open Reduction', *Ibid.*, **26**, 516.

Plastic and Maxillo-facial Trauma Symposium (1969), ed. GEORGIADE, N. G. St. Louis: Mosby.

QUINN, J. H. (1968), 'Open Reduction and Internal Fixation of Vertical Maxillary Fractures', *J. Oral Surg.*, **26**, 167.

ROBERTS, A., and others (1973), 'Prognosis of Odontoid Fractures', *Acta orthop. scand.*, **44**, 21.

ROBERTS, W. R. (1964), 'Case for Mandibular Plating', *Brit. J. oral Surg.*, **1**, 200.

ROBERTSON, J. H. (1963), 'Treatment of Fractures of Maxilla and Mandible by Resin Cap Splints', *Brit. dent. J.*, **114**, 321.

ROBINSON, M. (1959), 'Diagnosis of Mandibular Fractures by Auscultation with Percussion', *Oral Surg.*, **12**, 173.

— — (1960), 'New Onlay–inlay Metal Splint for the Immobilization of Mandibular Fractures', *Plastic reconstr. Surg.*, **25**, 77.

— — and YOON, C. (1963), ' "L" Splint for the Fractured Mandible: A New Principle of Plating', *J. oral Surg.*, **21**, 395.

— — and others (1963), 'Sleeve over Interosseous Wire to aid Immobilization of Jaw Fractures', *Plastic reconstr. Surg.*, **32**, 557.

ROBINSON, M. E. (1971), 'Delayed Surgical-occlusal Treatment of Malocclusion and Pain from Displaced Subcondylar Fractures: Report of Case', *J. Am. dent. Ass.*, **83**, 639.

ROWE, N. L. (1960), 'Mandibular Joint Lesions in Infants and Adults', *Int. dent. J., Lond.*, **10**, 484.

— — (1954), 'The Basic Principles of the Treatment of Maxillo-facial Injuries', *J. Roy. nav. Med. Serv.*, **40**, 111.

— — (1968), 'Fractures of the Facial Skeleton in Children', *J. oral Surg.*, **26**, 505.

— — (1969), 'Non-union of Mandible and Maxilla', *Ibid.*, **27**, 520.

— — and KILLEY, H. C. (1952), 'Fractures of the Facial Skeleton', *Dent. Practit.*, **3**, 34.

— — — — (1969), *Fractures of the Facial Skeleton.* Edinburgh: Livingstone.

SALEM, J., and others (1969), 'Analysis of 523 Mandibular Fractures', *Oral Surg.*, **26**, 390.

SAZIMA, H. J., and others (1971), 'Transoral Reduction of Mandibular Fractures', *J. oral Surg.*, **29**, 247.

SCHUCHARDT, K. N., SCHWENZER, B., ROTTKE, E. N., and LENTRODT, J. (1966), ' Ursachen, Häufigkeit und Lokalisation der Frakturen des Gesichtsschädels', *Fortschr. Kiefer- u. Gesichts-Chir.*, **11**, 1.

SCHULTZ, R. C. (1973), 'The Management of Common Facial Fractures', *Surg. Clin. N. Am.*, **53**, 3.

SHELTON, D. (1967), 'Study in Wound Ballistics', *J. oral Surg.*, **25**, 341.

SONG, I. C., and others (1965), 'Anterior Fixation of Mandibular Fractures', *Plastic reconstr. Surg.*, **35**, 317.

SOTHAM, J. C., and others (1971), 'Structural Changes around Screws used in the Treatment of Fractured Human Mandibles', *Brit. J. oral Surg.*, **8**, 211.

SPIESSL, B. (1972), 'Rigid Internal Fixation of Fractures of the Lower Jaw', *Reconstr. Surg. Traumatol.*, **13**, 124.

STONE, J. W., and others, 'Method of Bone Grafting the Mandible', *Sth. med. J., Nashville*, **65**, 815.

TAYLOR, D. V. (1966), 'Traumatic Aneurysm and Facial Palsy as Complications of a Mandibular Fracture', *Brit. J. oral Surg.*, **4**, 202.

THOMA, K. H. (1948), *Oral Surgery*, vol. 1. London: Kimpton.

— —(1951), 'Transosseous Wiring Fixation of Sub-condylar Fracture', *Oral Surg.*, **4**, 290.

— — (1959), 'Treatment of Jaw Fractures, Past and Present', *J. oral Surg.*, **17**, 30.

— — (1960), 'Progressive Atrophy of the Mandible complicated by Fractures: Its Reconstruction', *Oral Surg.*, **13**, 4.

THOMSON, H. G., and others (1964), 'Condylar Neck Fractures of the Mandible in Children', *Plastic reconstr. Surg.*, **34**, 452.

TREGGIDEN, R., WOOD, G., and BASHA, E. G. (1973), 'Traumatic Internal Carotid Artery Occlusion following Fracture of Mandible', *Brit. J. oral Surg.*, **11**, 25.

UPTON, L. G. (1971), 'Modified Healing in Experimental Mandibular Fractures', *J. oral Surg.*, **29**, 416.

VERO, D. (1968), 'Jaw Injuries. The Use of Kirschner Wires to Supplement Fixation', *Brit. J. Oral Surg.*, **6**, 18.

WALKER, D. G. (1957), 'Mandibular Condyle: Fifty Cases demonstrating Arrest in Development', *Dent. Pract.*, **7**, 160.

WALKER, G., HARRIGAN, W., ROWE, N. L., and WALKER, R. (1969), 'Clinical Pathological Conference on Facial Trauma', *J. oral Surg.*, **27**, 575.

WALKER, R. V. (1960), 'Traumatic Mandibular, Condylar Fracture Dislocations. Effect on Growth in the Macaca Rhesus Monkey', *Amer. J. Surg.*, **100**, 850.

WILDE, N. J. (1958), 'Malreduction, Malposition and Malunion in Facial and Mandibular Fractures', *J. int. Coll. Surg.*, **30**, 192.

WILLIAMS, D. W. (1968), 'A Modification of the Eyelet Wire', *Brit. J. oral Surg.*, **6**, 90.

YRASTORZA, J. A., and KRUGER, G. O. (1963), 'Polyurethane Polymer in the Healing of Experimentally Fractured Mandibles', *Oral Surg.*, **16**, 978.

ZAMBITO, R. F., and LASKIN, D. M. (1964), 'Follicular Cyst of Mandible associated with Pathologic Fracture', *J. oral Surg.*, **22**, 449.